High Blood Pressure

C000062940

Other titles in this series:
Candida Albicans
Irritable Bowel Syndrome
HRT and the Menopause

By the same author:
Candida Albicans
The Complete Book of Men's Health
Irritable Bowel Syndrome
HRT and the Menopause

Dr Sarah Brewer MA, MB, BChir

HIGH BLOOD PRESSURE

Thorsons
An Imprint of HarperCollins*Publishers*

Thorsons
An Imprint of HarperCollins*Publishers*
77–85 Fulham Palace Road,
Hammersmith, London W6 8JB
1160 Battery Street,
San Francisco, California 94111–1213
Published by Thorsons 1997

10 9 8 7 6 5 4 3

© Dr Sarah Brewer 1997

Dr Sarah Brewer asserts the moral right to
be identified as the author of this work

A catalogue record for this book
is available from the British Library

ISBN 0 7225 3390 X

Printed and bound in Great Britain by
Clays Ltd, St Ives plc

To Richard and Saxon

CONTENTS

PREFACE: THE ESSENTIAL GUIDE SERIES

This series offers up-to-date, in-depth information on common health problems. These books contain detailed, medically accurate information in a user-friendly, easy to read style.

Each book covers:

- What the condition is
- How common it is
- Who is affected by it
- Normal body functions and how each condition affects them
- Symptoms
- Causes
- Risk factors
- How the condition is diagnosed – blood tests, investigations, etc.
- Other similar conditions that need to be ruled out
- The drugs used to treat it – including side-effects and who shouldn't take them
- Surgical treatments that can help
- Complementary treatments
- Self-help tips
- Dietary changes that may prove helpful
- Latest research findings
- Addresses of support groups and sources of further information

This invaluable series will answer all your questions and help you to make the best decisions regarding your own health care.

chapter one

AN INTRODUCTION TO HIGH BLOOD PRESSURE

To keep blood moving around the body, everyone needs a certain pressure within their arteries. This is known as blood pressure (BP).

The best way to explain how your blood pressure is maintained is to compare circulating blood with water running through a hose pipe. Water pressure within a hose pipe can vary from high to low, depending on a number of factors. It can be raised by increasing the power of the pump (tap) or by squeezing the pipe and reducing its diameter. In exactly the same way, your blood pressure can be increased within the arteries by increasing the work of your heart (as through exercise) or by reducing the diameter of the vessels through which the blood flows (by, for example, the hardening and furring up of the arteries).

Your BP varies naturally throughout the day – it is lowest during sleep and highest from just before you wake until around three or four hours later. Your BP also goes up and down in response to lifestyle factors, including your emotions and level of activity.

If your BP temporarily falls too low (for example if you stand up suddenly) your brain may not receive enough blood to provide all the sugar and oxygen it needs, and you may feel dizzy or faint.

If your BP temporarily goes very high (such as after strenuous exercise) you will usually notice very little in the way of symptoms, although a few people develop a pounding sensation in their ears or develop a splitting headache.

If your blood pressure stays high all the time, even when you are at rest, your health is at risk. Constant high blood pressure is known as **hypertension** and is one of the most important conditions your doctor will ever screen you for.

HIGH BLOOD PRESSURE

High blood pressure is known as 'the silent killer' as it usually creeps up without any symptoms. If left untreated, it can lead to a sudden heart attack or stroke. Even if your blood pressure is dangerously high, you may feel relatively well. Because of this, it's worth having your blood pressure checked on a regular basis.

Who Gets High Blood Pressure?

High blood pressure is common. It affects as many as one in five adults, with more men affected than women. Blood pressure naturally tends to rise with age, so that hypertension is more common in middle life and beyond – some people, especially males, can develop it in their twenties or earlier, however. Blood pressure is also known to vary with race – those of African origin tend to have higher blood pressures than Caucasians, for example.

What Causes High Blood Pressure?

In most cases of hypertension there is no obvious single cause. This is referred to as primary, idiopathic, or essential hypertension. In 10 per cent of cases, an identifiable cause such as kidney problems, a hormone imbalance or drug side-effects is discovered. The high blood pressure is then referred to as secondary hypertension.

Several factors are thought to be involved in the development of essential hypertension. These include inherited factors (high blood pressure runs in some families), developmental factors (occurring during embryonic life in the womb) and environmental factors such as diet and lifestyle.

One of the main causes of hypertension is hardening and narrowing of the arteries. This naturally occurs with increasing age and comes on more quickly if you smoke or are overweight. Other environmental factors that can raise your blood pressure include obesity, eating too much salt, drinking too much alcohol, stress (in some people) and lack of exercise.

WHY HIGH BLOOD PRESSURE AFFECTS YOUR HEALTH

If your blood pressure remains consistently high, blood is forced through your system under high pressure. This over-stretches your arteries and damages blood vessel linings to such an extent that, if left untreated, it triggers hardening and furring up of the arteries. This can lead to a number of common health problems, including:

- angina (heart pain) or a heart attack – when the excess workload on the heart increases its oxygen and nutrient needs beyond those provided by the blood supply. This can happen as a result of, for example, narrowed coronary arteries
- cardiac failure – when your heart finds it difficult to pump blood against the high pressure in your circulation
- pulmonary oedema – a build-up of fluid in your lungs due to poor pumping action of the heart
- a stroke – if blood vessels in your brain are damaged
- failing sight – when blood vessels in your eyes are affected
- kidney failure – when blood vessels in your kidneys are damaged
- peripheral vascular disease – when the blood supply to your limbs is affected
- impotence – when the blood supply to the penis is affected.

This all sounds rather frightening – especially when it is estimated that half of all people with high blood pressure are undiagnosed, and of those that are picked up and treated, at least another half do not have acceptable blood pressure control. This is mostly because the condition rarely makes you feel ill – and having to take one, two or even three different types of tablet per day to treat something that is not an illness, but a risk factor for other diseases, is understandably frustrating. Early diagnosis and successful treatment of blood pressure will help to keep you healthy. You can also make relatively simple dietary and lifestyle changes that will reduce your risk of high blood pressure – and bring your BP down if it is already raised. Losing as little as 3–4 kg/half a stone in weight can be enough to bring a moderately raised blood pressure down to normal levels again, for example.

If your blood pressure is found to be high, you will have to have it measured several times before your doctor decides whether or not to prescribe any anti-hypertensive drugs. This is to make sure your blood pressure remains consistently high and is not just going up as a result of going to the surgery. Once you start taking blood pressure treatment, you may be on it for life – but you will probably live longer as a result.

chapter two

NORMAL CIRCULATION

Blood pressure exists because your heart pumps blood around a closed system. The pressure in your arteries is the product of how hard the heart pumps (cardiac output) and the elasticity or 'give' (peripheral resistance) of the blood vessel network. It also depends upon the volume of fluid inside your circulation, which varies to some extent as water and salts pass in and out of your smallest blood vessels (capillaries) to circulate through your tissues or to be filtered through the kidneys.

THE PUMP: YOUR HEART

Your heart is a fist-sized muscular organ that acts as a double pump. It has two sides, a right and a left, separated from each other by a thick, muscular wall known as the septum. Each side of your heart is made up of two chambers:

1. an upper atrium
2. a lower ventricle.

These chambers contract and relax around 70 times a minute at rest to keep blood flowing round your body. The atria only have to pump blood into the ventricles. The ventricles have to pump blood into the lungs or out into the body, against considerable pressure. The ventricles, therefore, have thicker, more muscular walls than the atria. Each of the four chambers holds exactly the same volume, however (70–90 ml).

The Route of Blood Flow

Several large arteries and veins are plumbed into your heart to transport blood to the atria, or away from the ventricles. Vessels bringing blood to the heart are called veins. Those taking blood away from the heart are called arteries.

Spent blood from your body, which contains little oxygen but lots of the waste gas carbon dioxide, arrives back at the heart – via your veins (venous system) – into the right atrium. From here, it is immediately pumped out into the larger, more muscular right ventricle and powered towards the lungs through the pulmonary artery.

In the lungs, blood passes through a series of small capillaries where waste carbon dioxide is off-loaded for excretion, and oxygen is taken on board for transportation around the body. Oxygenated blood then flows back into the heart through the pulmonary vein to arrive at the left atrium. The left atrium pumps blood into the most muscular chamber of all, the left ventricle, which pumps it out into general circulation through your largest artery, the aorta. You therefore have two main blood circulations:

1. the pulmonary (lung) circulation, which pumps blood from the right side of your heart to the lungs and back to the left atrium – this is a low-pressure system
2. the systemic circulation, which pumps oxygenated blood from the left side of your heart to the rest of your body, then back to the right atrium – this is a high-pressure system.

Blood flow through your heart is maintained in one direction by your four heart valves – the tricuspid, bicuspid, pulmonary and aortic valves. These open to let blood through, then close to prevent back-flow so blood keeps moving in the right direction.

Cardiac Output

Your cardiac output is the amount of blood pumped through your heart over a certain period of time. The amount of blood pumped out of each ventricle with each heart beat is around

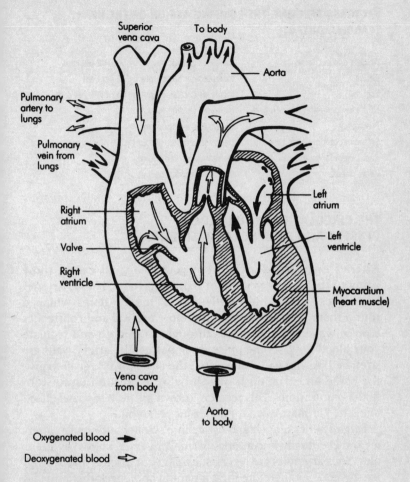

Figure 1: The heart

70 ml. In a resting man of average size, the heart beats around 72 times per minute, which means his cardiac output averages around 5L/min (70 ml × 72 beats/min = 5.04 L/min).

If cardiac output increases, more blood is pumped into the systemic circulation per minute, which increases blood pressure. If cardiac output falls, blood is pumped through the circulation more slowly and blood pressure falls.

FACTORS AFFECTING THE PUMPING ACTION OF THE HEART (CARDIAC OUTPUT)

Anxiety and excitement	Increases cardiac output by 50–100 per cent
Eating	Increases cardiac output by 30 per cent
Exercise	Increases cardiac output by up to 700 per cent
High environmental temperature	Increases cardiac output
Pregnancy	Increases cardiac output
Sitting or standing from lying	Decreases cardiac output by 20–30 per cent
Rapid irregular heart beat	Decreases cardiac output
Heart disease	Decreases cardiac output

THE CIRCULATION: YOUR BLOOD VESSELS AND PERIPHERAL RESISTANCE

Arteries carry blood away from your heart; all except those going to the lungs carry bright red, oxygenated blood. Arteries have thick, elastic walls with smooth muscle fibres wrapped round them. The arteries can therefore expand and contract as a pulse wave of blood passes through, to smooth and regulate your blood flow. As the pulse wave passes, the artery walls are stretched. As the wave moves on, the elastic walls recoil to give the blood an extra 'push' which helps to ensure that forward flow is continuous. This recoil is known as the *Windkessel* effect, after the German word for an elastic reservoir.

Large arteries branch and divide into smaller and smaller arteries and eventually into a series of smaller vessels known as arterioles. Your arterioles are less elastic than your arteries and are also narrower. They therefore form a natural bottleneck that provides more resistance to blood flow; they are known as resistance vessels. It is this resistance – against which your heart has to pump – that helps to maintain the blood pressure within your circulation. Factors that trigger constriction of arteries and arterioles (such as stress, emotion, smoking, taking certain drugs) will increase the peripheral resistance further and cause your BP to rise.

The arterioles connect up with a vast network of thin-walled blood vessels known as capillaries. Capillaries are the site where oxygen and nutrients pass from the bloodstream into the tissues,

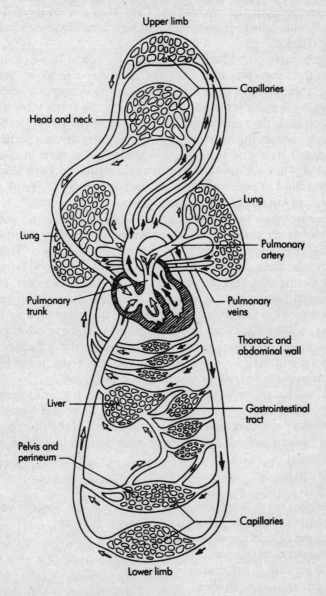

Figure 2: The circulatory system

while fluid and other substances – including wastes – pass from the tissues into the circulation. Capillaries are connected to small veins called venules, which in turn feed blood into larger vein trunks.

Veins carry blood back to the heart; all except those coming from the lungs carry dark wine-red, deoxygenated blood. Veins have thinner walls than arteries as the blood pressure within them is lower. Valves scattered throughout the larger veins help to stop back-flow and keep blood moving in the right direction – back towards the heart. Your veins are normally in a partially collapsed state and have an oval shape when seen in cross-section. They are capable of distending significantly to absorb excess fluid in order to even out fluctuations in BP. Veins are therefore known as capacitance vessels.

During exercise, the contraction of skeletal muscles compresses veins in the limbs and provides a secondary pumping action that helps to keep blood flowing through them. This is known as the muscle pump. It is so efficient that blood flow in contracting muscle is increased by as much as 30 per cent. Pulsation of nearby arteries may also compress the veins to keep blood moving forwards – back-flow is only prevented by the valves scattered throughout the larger veins. If these valves give way, blood may pool in certain veins under the influence of gravity, and may for example form varicose veins in the legs, scrotum (varicocoele), or rectum (haemorrhoids).

BP within the capillaries, venules and veins remains relatively constant, with a low pulse pressure of only around 5 mmHg. As blood flows back into the chest, the action of the rib cage on breathing in and out also helps to draw venous blood towards the heart.

At rest:

- 50 per cent of circulating blood volume is in the systemic veins
- 20 per cent in the pulmonary (lung) circulation
- 12 per cent in the chambers of the heart
- 2 per cent in the aorta
- 10 per cent in other arteries
- 5 per cent in capillaries
- 1 per cent in the arterioles.

The pulsatile delivery of blood to the body seems to be important for tissue health, although researchers do not know why. If an organ is perfused with blood by means of a pump delivering a constant, no-pulsed blood supply, the blood vessels in the organ gradually become hardened, their resistance goes up, and delivery of blood to the cells falls off.

- The circulatory system contains around 90,000 miles (150,000 km) of blood vessels.
- The circulation contains around 5 litres of blood.
- The aorta is the largest artery in the body and the vena cava is the largest vein.
- The heart pumps the equivalent of 13,640 litres of blood per day.
- The pulse wave of blood in the aorta travels at the rate of 120 cm/second.
- Blood moves through the capillaries quite slowly (0.07 cm/second), so that it takes a blood cell 1–2 seconds to pass through an average-sized capillary.
- Blood flows through the great veins at an average rate of 10 cm/second.

SYSTOLIC AND DIASTOLIC BLOOD PRESSURE

The contraction of your left ventricle, which pushes a volume of blood out into your circulation, causes a surge in your blood pressure with each heart beat. The highest pressure reached in your arteries during this surge is known as the systolic blood pressure, as it is due to contraction (systole) of your heart. As the heart rests between beats, blood pressure falls again to its baseline value. The lowest blood pressure recorded while the heart rests (diastole) is known as the diastolic pressure.

In general, a rise in cardiac output increases systolic pressure, while a rise in peripheral resistance increases diastolic pressure.

How Blood Pressure Is Measured

Blood pressure (BP) is measured using an instrument called a sphygmomanometer. This has an inflatable cuff which goes around your upper arm, a small pump to push air into the cuff and a column of mercury (or a dial) to record the pressure within the cuff.

As the cuff is inflated with air, the person measuring your BP usually palpates (feels with their finger for) your brachial pulse in the crook of your elbow. While the pressure within your artery stays higher than that in the cuff, blood can be felt pulsing through. Once the pressure in the cuff becomes greater than that in your artery, the vessel is squashed flat and blood stops flowing through it at that point. By inflating the cuff to an initial pressure that is higher than the expected systolic pressure, then listening with a stethoscope over your brachial artery as the pressure is slowly released, the point at which blood manages to squirt through again with each pulse can be heard distinctly as a tapping sound. The pressure registering in the blood pressure cuff at this point is taken as your systolic BP. The cuff is then slowly deflated further while listening over your artery. The tapping sounds become louder, then change to a dull whooshing sound before disappearing altogether. The point at which blood can no longer be heard whooshing through the vessel is taken as your diastolic BP.

Previously, some doctors preferred to record the diastolic BP as the point at which the arterial sounds suddenly became whooshing in nature, before actually disappearing. This was a less easy end-point to determine and resulted in a slightly higher diastolic pressure being recorded – by international convention, the disappearance of all sound in the vessel is now used.

BP is measured according to the length of a column of mercury it can support. Blood pressure is therefore expressed in millimetres of mercury (mmHg). BP is written down as the higher pressure (systole) over the lower figure (diastole), for example:

- A typical 20 year old will have a BP of around 120/70 mmHg.
- BP naturally tends to rise with age, so a fit 50 year old may have a BP of around 150/85 mmHg.
- The pulse pressure – the difference between the systolic and diastolic pressures – is normally around 50 mmHg.

- If your BP is consistently higher than 160/95, then you are suffering from high blood pressure, or hypertension.
- Blood pressure in the pulmonary (lung) circulation is low – such as 25/10 mmHg or less in the pulmonary artery.

YOUR FLUID BALANCE

Sixty per cent of your body weight is made up of water. Two thirds of this water is found inside your cells (intracellular), while the remaining third is found outside your cells (extracellular) in the so-called 'internal sea'. This extracellular fluid is divided up into the fluid that bathes your cells (interstitial fluid) and the fluid that circulates in your bloodstream (plasma) and which contributes to your blood pressure. Water molecules constantly pass from one fluid compartment to another as nutrients and waste substances are passed to and from your cells.

Your body normally maintains a tight fluid balance. During an average day in a temperate climate, you will lose a total of around 2.4 litres of fluid through your lungs as water vapour, your skin as sweat and through your kidneys as urine. A small amount is also lost in your bowel motions. If you take vigorous exercise or visit a hot climate, it is easy to lose twice this amount. However, as long as you replace your daily water losses through adequate drinking and eating, the amount of fluid in your cells, interstitial fluid and bloodstream is kept within narrow limits. Excess fluid passes into your circulation and is quickly filtered out by your kidneys. If you drink more fluid than you need, you will void increased amounts of urine. If you are slightly dehydrated, you will pass less urine than normal as your body carefully conserves its water stores and also triggers sensations of thirst.

If the fluid balance of the body becomes disturbed, excess water may stay in the interstitial fluid bathing your cells rather than passing into your bloodstream. This leads to water retention and puffiness, known as oedema. If excess fluid finds its way into your bloodstream, your blood pressure is not affected initially as the veins become distended and 'mop up' the extra fluid, becoming more and more distended until the point where BP starts to go up. Similarly, if you lose excessive amounts of water for any reason, the veins can collapse to a certain extent to protect the pressure in the system. If fluid loss from the circulation is excessive, however (as in the case of a haemorrhage), your BP will go down and you will develop what is known as clinical shock.

A 70-kg man contains:
- a total of 42 litres water:
- 28 litres within body cells (intracellular)
- 14 litres outside body cells (extracellular)
- of this, 10–11 litres are bathing the cells (interstitial fluid) and 3–4 litres are in the circulation.

HOW BLOOD PRESSURE IS NORMALLY CONTROLLED

Your blood pressure is normally controlled and kept within safe limits by a number of factors, including:

- alteration of the pumping action of your heart (cardiac output)
- changes in the diameter of your resistance vessels (mainly the arterioles)
- alterations in the amount of blood pooled in your capacitance vessels (veins)
- variations in the amount of salt and fluids in your circulation.

These factors are controlled by nerve signals from the brain, and by hormones or related substances released from various parts of the body including the kidneys (renin), the adrenal gland (aldosterone, adrenaline), pituitary gland (anti-diuretic hormone) and even the heart (atrial natriuretic peptide).

Baroreceptors

Your body monitors your blood pressure with special structures called baroreceptors found in the walls of the heart and at strategic blood vessels throughout your circulation. These respond to the degree of stretch your artery or vein walls are under. At normal blood pressures, they fire at a slow rate. If blood pressure falls, they discharge at an even lower rate, and if your blood pressure rises, they are stimulated at an increased rate. This sends signals to the brain that trigger a reflex:

- slowing or speeding up of your pulse rate and cardiac output
- dilation or constriction of blood vessels
- and a resultant decrease or increase in blood pressure until it returns to its previous normal level.

The baroreceptors in the heart are also part of a reflex that regulates the volume of water in your bloodstream and in the extracellular fluid bathing your tissues. By altering the amount of anti-diuretic hormone, renin and aldosterone produced, your kidneys retain varying amounts of fluid and salts to help maintain a relatively constant blood pressure.

The Renin-Angiotensin System

The most important hormone system that helps to control your blood pressure is known as the renin-angiotensin system.

Your kidneys produce a hormone, renin, which passes into the bloodstream and triggers a series of reactions that put your blood pressure up. This series of reactions starts when renin acts on a large sugar-protein molecule in the circulation known as *angiotensinogen*, or *renin substrate*. This molecule is made by the liver and circulates in the bloodstream until it meets up with renin. Renin splits angiotensinogen into two to release a small chain of 10 amino acids (protein building blocks) known as angiotensin I.

Angiotensin I is inactive, but as it travels around in the circulation it is acted on by an enzyme found in the cells lining your blood vessels. This enzyme, angiotensin converting enzyme (ACE) cuts a further two amino acids away from angiotensin I to form a chain of eight amino acids known as angiotensin II. This in turn is acted on by other enzymes (together known as angiotensinase) to produce angiotensin III.

Angiotensin II makes arterioles constrict and is one of the most powerful vasoconstrictors known. It rapidly produces a rise in both systolic and diastolic blood pressures. It also:

- acts on the brain to trigger a rise in BP, cause feelings of thirst and increase the secretion of anti-diuretic hormone (see below).
- acts on the adrenal glands to increase secretion of a hormone called aldosterone (see below).

All these actions work to increase the amount of fluid in the circulation and to produce a rise in blood pressure.

Angiotensin III has similar actions to angiotensin II but is only 40 per cent as powerful in boosting blood pressure.

High blood pressure can be treated by drugs that interfere with the action of angiotensin converting enzyme (ACE). These drugs are called ACE-inhibitors (*see Chapter 8 on Treatment*). Drugs called beta-blockers also work partly by decreasing renin secretion.

RENIN SECRETION

The release of renin is the body's way of quickly putting your blood pressure up. Its secretion is therefore boosted under certain circumstances, including:

- low blood pressure which is detected by receptors (baroreceptors) in the kidney
- lack of sodium
- treatment with diuretics
- haemorrhage
- standing upright
- dehydration.

It is also triggered by diseases such as constriction of the renal artery, heart failure, and cirrhosis of the liver.

Some forms of high blood pressure may be linked to over-secretion, or over-sensitivity to, renin or the angiotensins.

Anti-diuretic Hormone

Anti-diuretic hormone (ADH – also known as vasopressin) is one of the hormones secreted by the pituitary gland at the base of your brain. It acts to lower urine production in the kidney. This maintains the level of fluid in your circulation and helps to keep your BP up if, for example, you are dehydrated or have suffered a haemorrhage. It works by increasing the permeability of urine-collecting ducts in your kidney so that water in the urine which would otherwise have drained away as waste can be reabsorbed into the body. It is the effects of this hormone that make your urine increasingly concentrated (darker in colour and lower in volume) when you haven't drunk enough fluids. Some forms of high blood pressure may be linked to over-secretion, or over-sensitivity to, anti-diuretic hormone.

Aldosterone

Aldosterone is a steroid hormone produced in small amounts by your adrenal glands. It acts to increase reabsorption of sodium (in exchange for potassium) from the urine, sweat, saliva and intestinal juices to conserve your stores of sodium. This in turn draws water back into your body and plays a role in maintaining blood pressure. As sodium ions are swapped for potassium ones, the overall effect is a rise in sodium levels and BP, and a fall in potassium levels.

One form of secondary hypertension is due to over-secretion of aldosterone (primary aldosteronism due to an adrenal gland tumour).

The Effect of Gravity

Gravity also acts on blood in your system so that the average pressure in any vessel below heart level is increased, while the pressure in any vessel above heart level is decreased. For an adult human in the upright position, if the average arterial blood pressure at heart level is 100 mmHg, the average pressure in a large artery in the head is 62 mmHg, while the average pressure in a large artery in the foot would be 180 mmHg (the scientific formula to work this out is: density of blood × acceleration due to gravity × vertical distance above or below the heart).

Where pressure in the neck veins is close to zero, the vessels collapse so that pressure does not become sub-atmospheric (that is, less than the atmospheric pressure surrounding your body). Large venous spaces that surround the brain in the skull (dural sinuses) have a rigid structure and cannot collapse, however. The pressure in them while you are standing or sitting is therefore sub-atmospheric – sometimes by as much as minus 10 mmHg. When you stand up suddenly from a lying position, blood pressure in vessels taking blood to the brain falls and blood also starts to pool in your lower veins such as those in your legs. Without a safety mechanism to prevent blood flow to the brain decreasing, you would quickly faint on standing up. The sudden fall in blood pressure detected by baroreceptors in your heart and in the carotid artery in your neck triggers a reflex increase in cardiac output, constriction of arterioles, dilation of blood vessels within the brain, and a prompt increase in circulating levels of renin and aldosterone. These quick responses help to maintain blood pressure so that cerebral blood flow only decreases by around 20 per cent on standing, rather than the expected 60 per cent or more, which would quickly make you black out.

As long as you keep moving while standing, there is no further problem as the muscular pump action of your legs would help to keep blood flowing from the lower half of your body back to the heart. Prolonged standing still, however (such as undertaken by the guards outside Buckingham Palace!) can result in fainting due to pooling of blood in your lower veins due to the effects of gravity. Fainting is in fact a protective mechanism, as by falling down, you lie flat so that blood flow to the brain is restored.

Some people are very sensitive to sudden standing and can feel dizzy or faint, with a buzzing in their ears and spots before their eyes. This is called postural hypotension (low blood pressure related to body position) or orthostatic pre-syncope (feeling faint as a result of standing upright) and is common in the elderly and in people taking drugs to lower high blood pressure.

chapter three

HIGH BLOOD PRESSURE

Normal blood pressure (BP) varies naturally throughout the day, going up and down in response to your emotions and level of activity. If you have high blood pressure (hypertension), however, your blood pressure will remain high all the time, even when you are at rest. The World Health Organization defines hypertension as a blood pressure that is consistently greater than 160 mmHg (systolic) and 95 mmHg (diastolic). A systolic blood pressure of 140 to 160 mmHg and diastolic values of 90–95 mmHg are sometimes referred to as mild, or borderline hypertension.

As many as one in five adults suffers from hypertension. It is more common in men than women and is more likely in middle to old age. Surveys suggest that as many as 13 per cent of men and 11 per cent of women have a BP above 160/95 mmHg but are not receiving treatment for their condition.

Hypertension is not a disease in itself, but a clinical sign that you are at increased risk of a number of serious health problems such as coronary heart disease (CHD), stroke and heart or kidney failure. Research shows that for a man in his forties:

- each rise in systolic blood pressure of 10 mmHg increases his risk of heart disease by a massive 20 per cent
- the risk of having a stroke is 30 times higher than in someone with normal blood pressure
- reducing diastolic BP by as little as 5 mmHg would decrease the risk of CHD by as much as 16 per cent
- reducing average blood pressure by 10 mmHg would reduce the risk of premature death by a third.

WHAT ARE THE SYMPTOMS OF HIGH BLOOD PRESSURE?

High blood pressure is known as the silent killer. It usually creeps up on you without any warning, so that even if your blood pressure is dangerously high, you may feel relatively well. Most patients with high blood pressure don't notice any symptoms until their BP is severely raised. If symptoms do occur, they tend to be non-specific, such as a headache or having to get up at night to pass urine more often than normal. Your blood pressure has to be severely raised before you develop dizziness or visual disturbances.

THE CAUSES OF HIGH BLOOD PRESSURE

In chronic (long-term) hypertension, the baroreceptor reflexes that usually correct high or low blood pressure seem to be reset, so that your blood pressure is maintained at an elevated level compared to normal. Little is known about how or why this happens, but it seems to be readily reversible once lifestyle changes and/or drug treatment is started to treat the high blood pressure. Three main groups of factors can cause hypertension:

1. inherited factors
2. developmental factors
3. lifestyle factors.

Inherited Factors

In 90 per cent of cases, raised BP has no obvious cause; the condition is then described as primary, idiopathic, or essential hypertension. This is thought to be a result of inherited factors – genes – which may trigger high blood pressure as a result of any of a number of different mechanisms, or a combination of several abnormalities involving:

- sensitivity of the blood pressure monitors (baroreceptors) throughout the circulation
- altered secretion of, or sensitivity to, hormones or other factors (such as anti-diuretic hormone, renin, aldosterone) which help to regulate normal blood pressure
- dilation or constriction of blood vessels in response to blood pressure changes
- nerve control of BP or abnormal signals from the brain
- control of the amount of fluid and salt in the circulation
- control of cardiac output.

New research has identified a gene that may be able to predict your future risk of hypertension. People who have inherited the angiotensinogen gene (T235) from both parents have double the risk of developing high blood pressure and CHD than those who do not have the gene variant, or who only inherit it from one parent.

Developmental Factors

Fascinating new evidence suggests that the way you develop during the first few weeks of life as an embryo in your mother's womb affects your future risk of high blood pressure and other cardiovascular diseases in adult life. This is probably linked with lack of micronutrients in the maternal diet, which affects the way your arteries are laid down. Research suggests that:

- low birthweight babies are likely to develop high blood pressure as adults – average adult systolic BP increases by 11 mmHg as birthweight goes down from 3.4 kg (7.5 lb) to 2.5 kg (5.5 lb)
- the size of the placenta is also important – average systolic blood pressure rises by 15 mmHg as placental weight increases from 450 g (1 lb) to 680 g (1.5 lb) in weight
- the highest blood pressures therefore occur in men and women who were born as small babies with large placentas
- risk of high blood pressure in later life also increases:

- if a baby's birth length is small
- if the ratio of a baby's head circumference to the length of the baby is 0.7 or more
- if the mother's blood haemoglobin level is low during pregnancy
- if maternal nutrition is poor.

Lack of important nutrients – including vitamins, minerals and essential fatty acids – during the first few weeks of embryonic life is thought to trigger the development of abnormal arterial and blood circulatory patterns. These probably result due to an imbalance between the placenta and baby. This is supported by research linking fingerprint patterns with the risk of developing high blood pressure in later life. Fingerprints are laid down in the womb in the first few weeks following conception. Their patterns are linked to the degree of bumpiness and swelling of the developing fingertips, which is related in turn to irregular blood circulation.

Fingerprint patterns take the form of arches, loops or whorls; the more whorls you have, the more likely you are to become hypertensive in later life. Researchers have found that people with at least one whorl have a blood pressure that is 6 per cent higher (8 mmHg) than people with no whorls. BP, then, generally increases as the number of whorls increases, up to the maximum number possible, which is 10 (two per digit). The average number tends to be two or three overall. Long, narrow hands are also associated with higher blood pressure, and both effects are more marked with the right hand.

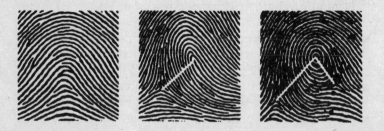

Figure 3: Fingerprint patterns

Lifestyle Factors

Inherited and developmental factors are not the whole cause of high blood pressure, however. Something else has to happen in any individual before blood pressure goes up, and this is where environmental or lifestyle factors come in. These environmental factors interact with inherited factors in individuals whose genes predispose them to hypertension to produce high blood pressure in later life. If several environmental factors linked with high blood pressure interact together, your risk of high blood pressure will be even greater. Fortunately, you can do something to address these factors and help lower high blood pressure.

Atherosclerosis

One of the main causes of high blood pressure – especially a raised systolic BP – is hardening and narrowing of the arteries (atherosclerosis). This naturally occurs with increasing age and comes on more quickly if you smoke or are overweight. High blood pressure in turn puts excessive strain on the arterial wall lining and triggers damage that hastens atherosclerosis. Because atherosclerosis in turn causes hardening of arterial walls, the blood vessels become less elastic and less able to distend to even out pressure surges, causing BP to rise even further. High blood pressure is therefore both a cause and a consequence of atherosclerosis, with each factor making the other worse (*see Chapter 5*).

Diabetes

Diabetes mellitus is a disease in which blood sugar (glucose) levels are raised due to lack of sufficient insulin hormone. Some people also have impaired glucose tolerance due to an inability of their cells to respond properly to relatively normal levels of insulin (insulin resistance). Having poorly controlled diabetes significantly increases the risk of developing atherosclerosis, high blood pressure, CHD and stroke – especially in women. The reason is not fully understood, but high blood sugar levels may trigger abnormal blood clotting, damage blood vessel linings (to trigger hardening and furring up), affect nerves controlling the heart and blood vessel function, or weaken muscles in the heart or artery walls.

Mortality rates from CHD are two to three times higher in men with diabetes, and three to seven times higher in women with diabetes, than in the general population. If you have high blood pressure and diabetes, it is vitally important that you keep your blood sugar levels under tight control. Keeping your weight within the healthy range and taking regular exercise will also help to prevent the type of diabetes that comes on in later life.

Smoking

Smoking greatly increases the risks associated with hypertension – people with high blood pressure who smoke are two or three times more likely to suffer from CHD than are hypertensive non-smokers; life insurance companies load their premiums accordingly. In the Western world, cigarette smoking is directly responsible for:

- 24 per cent of all male deaths from CHD
- 11 per cent of all female deaths from CHD
- 20 per cent of all deaths when cigarette-related cancers, stroke and chronic obstructive lung disease (such as chronic bronchitis, emphysema) are taken into account.

As a result:

- Smokers who die in middle age lose an average of 24 years of life.
- Smokers tend to die six years earlier than non-smokers.
- Cigarettes kill 40 per cent of smokers before they reach retirement.

Smoking cigarettes triggers hardening and furring up of the arteries (atherosclerosis) – as well as being linked with at least 90 per cent of all cancers. The reason that cigarette smoke is so noxious is that it contains chemicals which:

- damage the lining of arterial walls, triggering the build-up of clots and plaques which contribute to the hardening and furring up process (*see Chapter 5*)
- increase the stickiness of your blood, making serious blood clots (thrombosis) more likely
- displace oxygen from red blood cells in exchange for poisonous carbon monoxide – so that less oxygen is available for use by your tissues, including heart muscle cells
- trigger spasm of arteries all over your body, which increases blood pressure and decreases blood flow to vital areas such as the brain and heart
- produce harmful by-products of metabolism (known as free radicals) which damage tissues, increasing the risk of atherosclerosis and cancer.

Over 300 people die per day as a direct result of smoking and smoking-related diseases – as a result, doctors can now write 'smoking' as a cause of death on certificates.

Obesity

Obese people are more likely to have high blood pressure than thin people. Not everyone who is overweight has high blood pressure, as there is an interaction between obesity and some underlying, predisposing mechanism that is inherited by some people. In the UK, 38 per cent of men and 26 per cent of women are in the overweight range, and a further 13 per cent of men and 15 per cent of women are obese. Overweight is associated with an increased risk of hypertension because there is more peripheral resistance and a larger body tissue mass through which the heart has to pump blood. Overweight is also likely to result from an unhealthy diet with high intakes of saturated fat and raised blood fat levels, which in turn hasten the onset of atherosclerosis.

Overweight people also tend to be inactive. Lack of exercise means the heart is unfit, despite having to work extra hard to pump blood around the increased bulk of the body.

Where you store your excess fat is also important. Overweight people who carry excess weight around their middle (apple-shaped) rather than around their hips (pear-shaped) are at greater risk of CHD, stroke, high blood pressure, atherosclerosis, raised cholesterol levels and diabetes. The reasons are not fully understood, but may be linked to altered metabolism of dietary fats.

To work out your waist/hip ratio, measure your waist and hips in centimetres, then divide your waist measurement by your hip measurement. If the ratio is greater than 0.85 (women) or 0.95 (men), you are at increased risk of hypertension and CHD. You would be wise to make dietary and lifestyle changes to reduce your risk of future ill health (*see Chapter 10*).

Salt Intake

Sodium is the main positively-charged electrolyte found in the fluid bathing the outside of your body cells. A special salt pump in the cell membrane moves sodium out of your cells by swapping it for potassium, so your cells have a high potassium level inside them. This lets the cell act rather like a battery to maintain a small electric charge on its outer membrane. A certain amount of sodium is therefore essential for good health.

Researchers now believe that the rise in blood pressure seen with increasing age is directly linked to your lifetime's intake of excessive dietary salt (sodium chloride). In fact, some experts would say that hypertension developing in younger adults is just an early exaggeration of the sodium-induced rise in blood pressure that normally occurs with increasing age. Not everyone is sensitive to the effects of salt, however – there has to be an interaction between your salt intake and a genetic predisposition to hypertension. This interaction is as yet poorly understood. Researchers have just discovered a gene near the one for angiotensin converting enzyme (ACE) which they believe may increase your risk of inheriting salt sensitivity.

Ideally, you should obtain around 4–6 g salt (sodium chloride) per day from your diet. Average intakes are 9 g per day, with some people getting as much as 12 g daily – far too high. Unfortunately, as around 75 per cent of your salt intake is hidden in processed foods, it is not as easy as it sounds to reduce this amount.

Studies suggest that reducing salt intake by not adding salt during cooking or at the table can lower your systolic blood pressure by at least 5 mmHg. If everyone did this, it is estimated that the incidence of stroke in the population would be reduced by as much as 26 per cent, and CHD by 15 per cent.

Low Potassium Intake

Potassium is the main positively-charged electrolyte found inside your cells, where it balances the sodium ions found in your extracellular fluid. Potassium is essential for muscle contraction, nerve conduction and for the production of nucleic acids, proteins and energy. The main importance of potassium as far as blood pressure is concerned is that it helps to flush excess sodium out of the body through the kidneys – a special mechanism (a sodium-potassium pump) in the walls of the kidney tubules can swap a potassium ion for a sodium ion. Because the body swaps sodium for potassium in this way, a diet that is low in potassium is linked with a higher risk of high blood pressure and stroke – especially if your diet is also high in sodium.

Ideally, you need to obtain around 3,500 mg potassium per day. Most people get less than this, however, as the average intake is around 3,187 mg. Some people obtain as little as 1,700 mg potassium from their food. In general, fresh wholefoods – especially seafood, fruit and vegetables – are good sources of potassium and contain little sodium, while processed foods usually contain little potassium but lots of sodium (*see Chapter 10 for more on this*).

Alcohol

Another lifestyle factor linked with hypertension is drinking too much alcohol. People who regularly consume excessive amounts (more than 3 units of alcohol per day, or 21 units per week) tend to have higher blood pressure. Many people drink more than this and have a normal blood pressure, however – it depends on whether you have inherited predisposing factors for this and other lifestyle factors to act upon.

Lack of Exercise

Lack of exercise is an important cause of high blood pressure. People who exercise for at least 20–30 minutes three times per week have a lower risk of high blood pressure, stroke, obesity and CHD than those who are physically inactive. To be beneficial, exercise needs to be brisk enough to raise the pulse above around 120 beats per minute, to raise a light sweat and to make you slightly breathless.

Unfortunately, the average level of physical activity in the UK is low. Only 30 per cent of men and 20 per cent of women are active enough to gain some protection against high blood pressure. A recent survey among adult males found that one in five had taken no exercise at all during the preceding month. Although exercise increases cardiac output by up to 700 per cent and puts BP up during the period of exercise itself, this is a healthy, temporary response.

Taking regular exercise helps to fight high blood pressure by:

- burning off stress hormones that trigger arterial spasm in resistance vessels (mainly arterioles)
- dilating peripheral veins (capacitance blood vessels)
- increasing the efficiency of your cardiovascular system so your pulse rate falls
- boosting the muscle pump action of your skeletal muscles
- lowering blood fat levels
- reducing the risk of atherosclerosis.

Stress

High blood pressure is now thought by some researchers to be linked with excessive levels of stress in some people. Susceptible individuals have an overactive part of the nervous system (sympathetic nervous system) that is unusually responsive to stressful stimuli which would normally cause only a mild, temporary rise in blood pressure. This overactivity of sympathetic nerves is probably one of the inheritable factors that can run in families, with stress acting as the environmental factor that triggers the process off.

In people sensitive to stress, a condition known as Gaisbock's syndrome can occur. This is a form of hypertension in which blood pressure varies considerably from time to time, sometimes being high and sometimes low or normal. This can be a precursor to more permanent hypertension if your lifestyle doesn't slow down. One of the commonest signs of this is so-called

White Coat Hypertension – blood pressure that shoots up on being measured in the surgery or hospital. This can increase systolic BP by as much as 100 mmHg, although this is extreme. More commonly, White Coat Hypertension increases systolic BP by 20–30 mmHg. This form of hypertension is confirmed by attaching the sufferer to a 24-hour BP monitoring tape and showing that BP rises in stressful conditions, including having BP measured by a doctor, then falls again in between.

Until recently, White Coat Hypertension was thought to be relatively harmless. Latest research suggests that people with this condition should be treated with lifestyle changes and possible drugs. They have been shown to have just as many abnormalities of the heart and blood vessels (such as poor left ventricular function, decreased elasticity and increased stiffness of artery walls) as those with persistently high blood pressure. They are also likely to develop hypertension in the future.

In most people, however, stress only causes a transient rise in BP as a result of adrenaline hormone – this triggers constriction of arteries and veins, which temporarily puts blood pressure up. This is an adaptive response to help you fight or flee in dangerous situations. Blood pressure can still fall when you are at rest or asleep, which you will benefit from; relaxation training is also helpful in off-setting the effects of excessive stress.

Low Calcium Intake

Low intakes of calcium have recently been linked with an increased risk of high blood pressure and stroke. Your body contains more calcium than any other mineral. Ninety-nine per cent (around 1.2 kg) is stored in your skeleton (bones and teeth), while the other 1 per cent (around 10 g) plays a central role in the way your muscles contract, nerve conduction, blood clotting, the regulation of metabolic enzymes, energy production and immunity. Lack of calcium may affect the way your circulation responds to changes in blood pressure detected by your baroreceptors – perhaps by interfering with the nerve signals to arterioles which encourage them to dilate.

Drugs that affect calcium channels in the body are highly successful in treating hypertension, angina, some irregular heart rhythms and poor circulation. Low intakes of magnesium –

which works together with calcium in the body – may be a risk factor for hypertension, too. Increasing your intake of calcium and magnesium can help (*see page 145*).

Lead
Two recent studies have looked for a possible link between lead levels in the body and the development of high blood pressure or kidney damage. They found that men with the highest amount of lead in their bones have the greatest risk of hypertension and of developing poor kidney function. If these findings are correct, it may mean that lead has toxic effects on the heart, blood vessels or kidneys – hypertension could perhaps be a disease brought on by pollution.

Keloids
Interestingly, people who develop an excessive scar tissue reaction to a skin wound and produce a large, lumpy keloid scar seem to be twice as likely to develop high blood pressure in the future compared with people who produce normal amounts of scar tissue. This is thought to be due to the blood protein angiotensin II (*see page 15*), which helps to control blood pressure. It is now also known to stimulate the production of collagen – a fibrous protein found in scar tissue. A group of drugs that block angiotensin (angiotensin converting enzyme [ACE] inhibitors) are commonly used to treat high blood pressure. This link is currently the result of much research in an attempt to unravel some of the mysteries of essential hypertension.

Homocysteine
If you have hypertension, a new blood test may be able to predict your future risk of a heart attack or stroke. Men with high blood levels of a particular amino acid – homocysteine – are three times more likely to have a stroke or heart attack than men with low levels (similar data regarding women is not available, as men are more likely to have raised levels of homocysteine). Moderately raised levels of homocysteine are relatively common, with 10 per cent of men inheriting a genetic inability to metabolize this amino acid properly. As a result, it builds up in the circulation, where it is thought to damage blood vessel

linings, interfere with blood vessel dilation and encourage hardening and furring up of the arteries. One in 160,000 people has extremely high levels (a condition known as homocysteinuria) and 30 times the risk of premature cardiovascular problems.

To help discover those at risk, a new homocysteine test has been launched which can measure levels in the blood or urine. If your level is high, this can be reduced by taking supplements of the B group vitamins folic acid, B_6 and B_{12}. These vitamins are found in foods such as orange juice, broccoli, spinach, lettuce, bananas, baked potatoes, beef and fish, but many people fail to obtain enough from their diet. In the US, for example, only 40–50 per cent of people get enough folic acid; supplements of 400–650 mcg per day would be beneficial.

For more details of the homocysteine test, contact Larkhill Green Farm on 0181–874 1130.

How Environmental Factors Interact

More than one factor may be at work in any individual to increase his or her risk of hypertension. At the same time, several abnormal genes are probably involved, too. If you obtain excess dietary salt while you are under excess stress, for example, you are more likely to develop high blood pressure than if you just have too much salt, or are just under long-term stress.

MALIGNANT HYPERTENSION

Despite its name, malignant hypertension has nothing to do with cancer. It refers to the most dangerous type of high blood pressure in which pressures go very high, often very quickly. This can damage internal organs over a short period of time and is sometimes also referred to as accelerated hypertension. It is treated as a medical emergency, for if diastolic pressure remains above 120 mmHg for a prolonged period of time, the lining of small blood vessels (arterioles) are damaged and start to leak. When looked at under the microscope, the blood vessel walls have literally started to crumble (fibrinoid necrosis, *see Chapter 7*).

Treatment aims to bring BP down slowly over several days so that the body can adjust to lower pressures again.

To differentiate it from malignant hypertension, primary (idiopathic, essential) high blood pressure is often referred to as benign essential hypertension.

REFRACTORY HYPERTENSION

Refractory hypertension refers to high blood pressure that does not respond to standard first-line anti-hypertensive drug treatments. Although it is uncommon, referral to a specialist is needed so that investigations and treatment with other second-line drugs can be started.

ROUTINE EXAMINATION OF PEOPLE WITH HYPERTENSION

- checking your blood pressure at least twice during the first visit
- feeling your pulse to see how regular and strong it is
- checking pulses in your groin, feet and ankles to make sure your peripheral circulation is intact – pressing on the skin of your lower legs and then letting go will show how quickly blood flows back into the area
- feeling your chest to see where the tip of your beating heart is detectable – this gives a good indication of whether or not your heart is enlarged
- listening to your heart with a stethoscope to check for heart murmurs and to listen to your heart beat rhythm
- listening to your lungs to check for signs of fluid build-up on the chest
- listening to your neck and abdomen with a stethoscope to detect any noises due to turbulent blood flow through damaged carotid or renal arteries
- examining the backs of your eyes to look for any signs of arterial damage

ROUTINE SCREENING TESTS PERFORMED ON PEOPLE WITH HYPERTENSION

- chest x-ray to check the size and shape of the heart and to look for evidence of congestive heart failure with fluid build-up on the lungs
- ECG – to look for signs of left ventricular thickening, irregular heart beat or evidence that the heart muscle is struggling
- urinalysis – to look for protein and sugar
- fasting blood lipids – to see if your blood cholesterol or other fat levels are raised
- urea and electrolytes – to check kidney function and your salt balance.

Chapter Four

SECONDARY HYPERTENSION

In around 1 in 10 cases, hypertension is found to result from another illness or condition, in which case it is referred to as secondary hypertension. Secondary hypertension should always be ruled out in any hypertensive patient, but it is especially important to exclude other conditions in people developing high blood pressure before the age of 35.

The most common cause of secondary hypertension is kidney (renal) disease, which accounts for 8 out of 10 cases. The kidney diseases involved are:

- chronic glomerulonephritis (inflammation of the kidney filtration units)
- chronic atrophic pyelonephritis (shrinking of kidney tissue due to chronic infection or inflammation)
- congenital polycystic kidneys (abnormal kidney structure due to the formation of multiple cysts during embryonic life).

Kidney problems are thought to cause high blood pressure by triggering retention of fluid and salt, which builds up in the circulation and elsewhere in the body.

As high blood pressure in itself can cause kidney disease (see Chapter 7), it can sometimes be difficult for a doctor to work out if the renal problems caused the hypertension or vice versa.

Other relatively common causes of secondary hypertension include:

- pre-eclampsia during the last three months of pregnancy (which affects around 1 in 10 pregnant women – see below)
- the side-effects of some drugs.

Rarer causes of secondary hypertension include:

- anatomical abnormalities of the circulatory system such as an abnormally narrowed aorta (coarctation of the aorta) or renal artery (renal artery stenosis)
- polycythaemia (significantly increased blood stickiness due to over-production of red blood cells)
- Conn's syndrome (due to high levels of aldosterone hormone)
- phaeochromocytoma (due to a tumour that secretes excessive amounts of adrenaline hormone and noradrenaline)
- Cushing's syndrome (due to excessive exposure to corticosteroids – either from overactive adrenal glands or from steroid drug treatment)
- acromegaly (due to excessive production of growth hormone by the pituitary gland)
- hyperparathyroidism (due to overactivity of the four parathyroid glands in the neck, which if not treated raises blood calcium levels which can damage the kidneys).

SCREENING TESTS PERFORMED ON PEOPLE WITH SUSPECTED SECONDARY HYPERTENSION

- If your potassium level is low, and you are not on diuretic treatment, you may have a hormone problem leading to high blood pressure. You will therefore have blood tests taken to check levels of aldosterone, cortisol and renin.
- blood tests to assess kidney function (creatinine clearance rate)
- an intravenous urogram – a substance that shows up on x-ray is injected into your bloodstream and a series of x-rays taken. This shows any narrowing of your renal arteries, how well your kidneys concentrate the dye in the urine, and outlines your urinary system to show up anatomical abnormalities or shrinkage of the kidneys.
- ultrasound of your kidneys
- blood tests to measure catecholamine levels or measurement of urinary vanillylmandelic acid if phaeochromocytoma (tumour of the adrenal gland) is suspected
- acromegaly is usually obvious from changes to your features and the fact that your tongue, jaw, hands and feet are getting bigger – if this is suspected you will have your blood levels of growth hormone measured.

BLOOD PRESSURE AND PREGNANCY

Pregnancy is a time when blood pressure is often lower than normal due to changes in the circulation. While blood volume increases by as much as 30 per cent, increased production of progesterone hormone relaxes smooth muscles throughout the body – including those in the artery walls – so that blood vessels dilate more than enough to hold this extra fluid. As a result, BP usually goes down. If blood pressure increases during pregnancy, however, the sudden rise can:

- affect the function of the placenta so the baby doesn't grow as well as expected
- increase your risk of a miscarriage
- damage small arteries in your kidneys, leading to kidney problems
- damage small arteries in the brain, increasing your risk of an epileptic fit (eclampsia – see below) or a stroke.

A blood pressure above 140/90 is therefore considered high in a pregnant woman – especially if it develops for the first time during the pregnancy. If you have pre-existing high blood pressure, you may be advised to take anti-hypertensive medication to control your BP before you get pregnant. Once you conceive, you will need close supervision throughout the pregnancy to ensure that your BP doesn't go too high.

If your blood pressure is usually normal, but suddenly rises during pregnancy, this is a sign of pre-eclampsia.

Pre-eclampsia

Pre-eclampsia is one of the most common and serious complications of pregnancy. It usually comes on after the 20th week and results in three classic signs:

1. raised blood pressure (above 140/90)
2. fluid retention (such as puffy ankles and fingers)
3. leaking of protein into the urine.

It is more common in:

- a first pregnancy
- women under the age of 25
- those over 35
- those with a family history of pre-eclampsia
- women expecting twins or a multiple birth
- women with pre-existing diabetes, high blood pressure or kidney disease.

As many as 1 in 10 pregnant women suffer from pre-eclampsia (1 in 5 first-time mothers), with 50,000 women affected each year in the UK alone. Most cases are mild, but 1 in 20 first-time mothers suffer moderate pre-eclampsia, and 1 in 50 cases (1 in 25 first pregnancies) suffer pre-eclampsia that is severe enough to put the life of the mother and baby at risk. Sadly, at least seven women and 1,000 babies die from the condition every year in the UK. Most women with pre-eclampsia do not suffer a recurrence in future pregnancies – the risk of a severe recurrence is 1 in 20.

Why It Happens

The exact cause of pre-eclampsia is still unknown, but is thought to be linked with faulty development of the placenta. If placental arteries do not dilate properly, placental tissues become starved of oxygen. This may trigger release of an unidentified substance that affects the mother's circulation. Another theory is that pre-eclampsia is due to an over-zealous immune system. A developing baby contains foreign genes inherited from the father; pre-eclampsia may be a form of tissue rejection similar to that of a poorly-matched transplanted organ.

Unfortunately, pre-eclampsia does run in families. A woman whose sisters or mother were affected is six times more likely to develop it during her first pregnancy than a woman with no family history of the disease.

The Early Signs

Ante-natal tests are designed to detect pre-eclampsia early, before it does any harm. It is usually symptomless in the early stages, which is why ante-natal screening is important to pick up the early clinical signs of:

- rising blood pressure
- leaking of protein (albumin) into the urine
- retention of fluid leading to puffiness of the ankles, fingers or face – this does not always occur and can be difficult to tell apart from the normal swelling that commonly occurs during pregnancy, especially towards the end when the weight of the womb interferes with the return of blood from veins in the legs.

In the later stages of pre-eclampsia, headache, nausea and vomiting, abdominal pain and visual disturbances will occur, along with a tailing off of the baby's growth rate.

How It Is Treated

Pre-eclampsia is a progressive disease that can get worse as pregnancy continues.

Mild cases are usually controlled by strict bed rest. A woman with moderate pre-eclampsia will need admission to hospital and drugs to bring her blood pressure down.

In severe cases, early delivery is essential, either by inducing labour or by having a Caesarean section. This usually allows the mother's symptoms to resolve quickly. The baby's progress will depend on his or her age at delivery.

If you are told you have pre-eclampsia, it is vitally important that you attend all ante-natal appointments and follow the advice of your doctors and midwife. The health of both you and your baby is at stake. If left unchecked, pre-eclampsia can lead to organ damage, blood clotting disturbances, haemorrhage or fits. This serious condition is known as eclampsia. Eclampsia affects around 1 in 2,000 pregnant women and may be serious enough to cause maternal or fetal death.

SECONDARY HYPERTENSION DUE TO DRUGS

Several drugs – both those available on prescription and those bought over the counter – can put your blood pressure up while they are being taken. These include:

- nasal decongestants (such as ephedrine)
- non-steroidal anti-inflammatory drugs (such as ibuprofen) taken to relieve aches and pains in the muscles and joints, which can raise BP by 5–10 mmHg
- oral corticosteroids (taken for severe inflammatory conditions such as asthma or rheumatoid arthritis)
- the combined oral contraceptive pill (containing both oestrogen and progestogen hormones), which can raise BP after several years' use – recent research suggests that the average increase in BP is around 2.8/1.9 mmHg. In some women, however, rapid and more severe rises in BP can occur – which is why BP is checked regularly every six months in women taking the combined pill.
- monoamine-oxidase inhibitors – drugs sometimes used to treat severe depression – can cause sudden rises in BP if you eat cheese or other foods containing tyramine while on medication
- carbenoxolone – a synthetic version of liquorice, which is sometimes used to treat stomach ulcers – can put BP up as it can trigger retention of sodium and water. A similar effect can also occur if you eat too much liquorice.
- ginseng – there are three types: Korean ginseng (*Panax ginseng*), Siberian ginseng (*Eleutherococcus senticosus*) and American ginseng (*Ginseng quinquefolium*). Long-term use, especially if Korean ginseng, can put up blood pressure.

Chapter Five

HIGH BLOOD PRESSURE AND CORONARY HEART DISEASE

Coronary heart disease (CHD) is due to hardening and furring up of the coronary arteries. This causes narrowing of the vessels so that the heart muscle does not receive all the oxygen-rich blood it needs. CHD is the biggest killer in the Western world, killing more people than any other single disease. In the UK, it:

- accounts for around half of all deaths
- is responsible for 1 in 3 male deaths each year
- causes 1 in 4 female deaths each year
- kills 1 in 6 men prematurely (before the age of 75)
- kills 1 in 15 women prematurely.

Having uncontrolled high blood pressure significantly increases your risk of CHD in later life.

THE HEART'S BLOOD SUPPLY

The heart is made up of a special type of muscle (the myocardium) that beats continuously around 70 times per minute when you are at rest. Because of this constant activity, heart muscle needs much larger supplies of oxygen and nutrients than any other muscle in the body. Although the chambers of the heart are continuously being filled with blood as it is pumped round the circulation, oxygen and nutrients can only diffuse a little way into the heart's thick muscular walls. Your heart muscle is therefore directly supplied with blood from branches of the main artery (aorta) plumbed into your left ventricle. These vessels are known as the:

- left coronary artery
- right coronary artery.

As a general rule, your right ventricle is supplied with blood from the right coronary artery, your left ventricle via the left coronary artery, and the wall (septum) between the two sides of the heart by both coronary arteries. The blood supply to the two upper chambers of the heart (the atria) is more variable from person to person. As a constant supply of blood to your heart muscle is so important, the two coronary arteries join up in places to help safeguard against problems with blood supply from one or the other.

CORONARY HEART DISEASE

CHD occurs when the coronary arteries become narrowed or blocked. As a result, they cannot supply enough blood to meet the oxygen demands of your myocardium. Tissue that is not receiving enough oxygen is said to be *ischaemic*, and CHD is sometimes also referred to as ischaemic heart disease. Tissues that are ischaemic produce an intense pain, which in the case of heart muscle feels like a tight, crushing sensation behind the sternum (*see angina, below*).

If the inadequate blood supply continues, the oxygen-starved heart tissues suffer irreversible damage, and some cells die in a process known as infarction. When this happens to heart muscle (myocardium) it is referred to as myocardial infarction – otherwise known as a heart attack.

Like other arteries in the body, the coronary arteries have three layers:

1. a smooth, inner lining
2. a thick, muscular, elastic middle layer
3. a tough, fibrous outer coating.

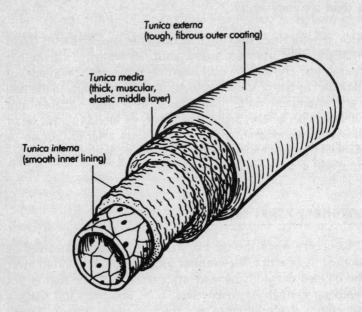

Figure 4: The three layers of the coronary arteries

Healthy arteries are elastic and, as described in Chapter 2, help to even out the peaks and troughs of blood pressure produced by the beating heart. Disease of the coronary arteries can lead to CHD in two main ways:

1. through furring up of the inner lining of a coronary artery with discreet plaques (atheroma) that cause narrowing
2. by hardening of the middle layer of a coronary artery (arteriosclerosis) with loss of elasticity and the ability to dilate.

These two processes usually occur together and are referred to as atherosclerosis – hardening and furring up of the arteries. This process is also both a cause of rising blood pressure and an effect of it, as high blood pressure causes arterial damage which hastens the hardening and furring up process.

Atherosclerosis

Atherosclerosis starts early in life, usually in the teens, and is triggered by normal wear-and-tear damage to your artery walls. Once the damage occurs, small cell fragments in the bloodstream – known as platelets or thrombocytes – stick to the damaged area and form a tiny clot. These platelets release chemical signals to stimulate healing of the damaged area. Under normal circumstances, this would lead to healing, but if excessive damage continues (as a result of high blood pressure, raised cholesterol levels or lack of antioxidants in the diet, for example), the damaged area becomes infiltrated with a fatty porridge-like substance that builds up to form a plaque (atheroma). When examined under the microscope, the fatty plaques are full of scavenger cells which have become stuffed full with globules of fat to the extent that they die and accumulate in the artery wall.

While the scavenger cells remain in the circulation, they are known as monocytes. Once they leave the bloodstream and enter the body tissues to pick up and destroy dead cells and debris, the scavenger cells are known as macrophages. New research into atherosclerosis suggests that CHD is a chronic inflammatory disease, as circulating blood monocytes only leave the bloodstream to take part in inflammation. The macrophages seem to be attracted into the artery walls by something coming from the environment – and the most likely culprits are dietary fats.

The most popular theory is that certain fats from the diet are taken up into the artery wall where circulating monocytes mistake them for invading bacteria. The monocytes leave the bloodstream and enter the artery wall in an attempt to engulf the fats and destroy them. The macrophages aim a cocktail of powerful chemicals against the fats and oxidize them, setting up an inflammatory reaction that attracts more macrophages into the area. The most harmful molecules come from oxidation of a type of fat called omega-6 polyunsaturated fatty acids (PUFAs).

Unlike saturated fats, polyunsaturated fatty acids have a molecular structure containing spare double bonds. This makes them highly reactive and more susceptible to chemical change, such as when oxidized by macrophages. This chemical change produces toxic substances known as lipid peroxides, which are now linked with hardening and furring up of artery walls (atherosclerosis).

There are two main types of polyunsaturated fat:

1. omega-3 PUFAs, mainly derived from fish oils
2. omega-6 PUFAs, mainly derived from vegetable oils.

Your body handles omega-3 and omega-6 oils in different ways. Omega-3 fish oils have a thinning effect on your blood and are good for the heart, while omega-6 PUFAs are increasingly thought to be linked with inflammatory processes in the body. The current idea is that increased levels of inflammatory diseases (such as CHD, asthma, rheumatoid arthritis, inflammatory bowel disease) are due to low intakes of omega-3 PUFAs and increased intakes of omega-6s. Saturated (animal) fats traditionally thought of as the 'baddies' when it came to CHD are now thought to be less important – especially if your intake of antioxidants is high (*see page 140*).

How Atherosclerosis Leads to CHD and High Blood Pressure

Untreated hypertension leads to atherosclerosis by damaging artery linings and hastening the hardening and furring up process. Once atherosclerosis is established, it also acts to raise your blood pressure and a vicious cycle sets in.

Once the initial damage has occurred, atheromatous plaques slowly build up and form fatty streaks along artery walls – including the coronary arteries supplying the heart muscle. Further damage to a plaque – which occurs slowly through normal wear and tear or more quickly due to smoking cigarettes or having hypertension – causes ulceration of the plaque surface. Extra platelets stick to the ulcerated area to form a larger clot (thrombus), and more macrophages are attracted into the area. This results in the typical layered build-up of clot and fatty substances which increasingly narrows the coronary arteries. Over a period of time, this causes a significant fall in blood supply to parts of the body. When one or more coronary arteries become narrowed with atheromatous plaques, heart muscle is at risk of lack of oxygen (ischaemia), especially when its workload and oxygen needs increase, as during exercise.

If atherosclerosis is widespread throughout the body, it narrows the circulation and causes the diastolic BP – the pressure in the system when the heart is at rest between beats – to be set at a higher level.

At the same time as atheromatous plaques are developing, the underlying middle layer of the artery wall is affected and starts to degenerate, becoming fibrous and much less elastic. This means that the peaks and troughs of blood pressure produced by the beating heart are not smoothed out, so the blood pressure shoots up higher when the heart contracts.

Atherosclerosis, therefore, raises both diastolic and systolic blood pressure. If left untreated, the raised BP in turn causes damage to the arterial system which hastens the development of atherosclerotic plaques, and blood pressure rises even further. As a result, the heart has to pump blood out into a circulation whose vessels are narrowed and have lost their elasticity. This increases the workload of the heart – as it has to pump blood out into a high-pressure system – and its need for oxygen, at a time when its blood supply is already compromised. As heart muscle beats over 100,000 times per day, lack of oxygen rapidly leads to muscle cramping, making angina and a heart attack more likely.

The Symptoms of CHD

Untreated high blood pressure is one of the major causes of CHD. Poor blood supply to the heart may cause no problems, but commonly triggers:

- heart pain (angina pectoris)
- heart attack (myocardial infarction or coronary thrombosis)
- irregular heart beat (arrhythmia)
- heart pump failure
- sudden death.

In some patients, two-thirds or more of a coronary artery may be furred up and blocked with atheroma without causing symptoms.

In others, angina may be triggered even though only a small atheromatous plaque is present and the coronary artery is only narrowed slightly. It all depends on:

- the exact site where the atheroma and narrowing have developed – the most common site is within 3 cm of where a coronary artery originates from the aorta, so that the effects of ischaemia are likely to be more widespread and serious
- how well the two coronary arteries join up (anastomose) to share the load of supplying blood
- how good the blood supply from the other coronary artery is
- the type of coronary arteries you have inherited – whether they are the vascular equivalent of motorways or winding country lanes.

ANGINA

Angina is the name given to the pain triggered by lack of oxygen to heart muscle (myocardium). This ischaemic pain is usually:

- felt behind the chest bone (retrosternal)
- tight and crushing – like a bear hug
- described as spreading through the chest and radiating up into the neck, jaw or down the left arm.

Almost 2 million people suffer from angina in the UK each year. The pain varies in intensity from person to person, and usually comes on when the heart is working harder than usual, such as during exertion such as walking uphill. This is known as 'effort angina' and usually stops after the sufferer rests.

A more serious form of ischaemic chest pain comes on at rest when the heart is not under increased strain. This implies that the blood supply to the heart is seriously impaired. Unlike effort angina, where each attack is usually similar to previous ones, pain coming on at rest tends to differ in frequency, duration and intensity. It is therefore known as unstable angina.

Patients with unstable angina are at a higher risk of suffering a heart attack. It may be due to:

- tiny platelet clots coming and going at the site of an atheromatous plaque, which intermittently block the blood supply to the heart
- arterial spasm which worsens an already poor blood supply to heart muscle.

Arterial spasm may in fact be involved in both types of angina. Spasm can be triggered by stress, by smoking a cigarette, by exercise or as part of an artery's normal dynamic activity.

HEART ATTACK

If an atherosclerotic plaque fractures, it will bleed into the artery wall. This triggers a rapid build-up of thrombocytes and the development of a clot which may be large enough to block the artery and suddenly cut off circulation to part of the myocardium. This causes a heart attack when heart muscle cells are so starved of oxygen that they suffer irreparable damage and die. In the UK, a heart attack – also known as a coronary thrombosis (literally, a clot in a coronary artery) or a myocardial infarction (literally, death of heart muscle due to lack of blood and oxygen) affects 330,000 people each year and kills 170,000 a year (nearly 500 people every day).

The pain of a heart attack is similar to that of angina in that it is tight, crushing and felt behind the sternum. It differs from angina in that it tends to:

- come on when the sufferer is at rest
- last longer
- be more intense
- be unrelieved by rest
- usually be accompanied by other symptoms: the sufferer becomes pale, sweaty, breathless, has an urge to open his or her bowels, or develops frightening feelings of impending doom.

Sudden chest pain should always be taken seriously and medical assistance sought without delay. If it is due to a heart attack, the first two hours are critical. If treatment can restore the blood supply to the damaged muscle by opening up a blocked coronary artery, the ischaemic heart tissue can be saved.

Sometimes, especially in the elderly, a heart attack may cause no pain and the patient may just complain of sudden tiredness or an irregular pulse, or (if suffering from heart pump failure) with breathlessness, swollen ankles, extreme tiredness and weight gain caused by fluid retention.

OTHER CHD RISK FACTORS

A risk factor is any characteristic that increases your susceptibility to an illness. If you suffer from uncontrolled high blood pressure, your risk of CHD increases if other risk factors are also present. Those most closely associated with hardening and furring up of the arteries and having a heart attack are:

- increasing age
- having a family history of heart disease
- smoking cigarettes
- being overweight or obese
- having abnormally raised blood fat (cholesterol and/or triglyceride) levels
- not taking exercise (sedentary lifestyle)
- having high stress levels
- drinking excessive amounts of alcohol
- having poorly controlled diabetes
- eating a diet that is low in antioxidants.

Too many people wait until they have had a first heart attack before tackling the risk factors they have some control over. If you suffer from high blood pressure, you should do something about your diet and lifestyle risks now – before they do something to you.

HEART FAILURE

Untreated hypertension is the commonest cause of heart failure, which affects as many as 1 in 10 people over the age of 65.

High blood pressure makes it difficult for the heart to pump blood out into the circulation against the resistance due to the increased pressure. As a result, the left ventricle starts to thicken (hypertrophy) just like any other muscle that is given extra work to do. Over many years, high blood pressure can lead to such pronounced thickening of heart muscle and dilation of the heart chambers that the heart becomes a floppy, dilated bag of muscle. It then cannot contract properly and the amount of blood it pumps (cardiac output) falls below that needed to meet the demands of the body. This is known as heart failure and refers to the inability of the heart to pump properly – it does not mean that the heart is about to stop suddenly.

Heart pump failure results in fluid accumulating within the body. Left-sided heart failure usually occurs first when high blood pressure is the cause. This means that less fluid is pumped from the lungs into the left ventricle and out into the aorta. This causes fluid to accumulate in the lungs, leading to increased shortness of breath during exertion or even when at rest. It can also stop sufferers lying flat at night, so that they have to prop themselves up with several pillows. This is known as orthopnoea. In some cases, it can make sufferers wake at night gasping for breath (paroxysmal nocturnal dyspnoea).

The backed-up pressure resulting from left-sided heart failure then puts extra strain on the right side of the heart, which may then start to fail, too. This means that less blood is pumped from the body into the right ventricle and on into the lungs. Fluid then pools in the legs under the influence of gravity. The first sign is usually swelling of the ankles. In severe cases, fluid may collect all the way up the legs and even around the buttocks and lower abdomen.

When both sides of the heart fail together, so that fluid accumulates in both the lungs and the legs, this is known as congestive cardiac failure.

The thickened heart muscle is also likely to outgrow its blood supply, increasing the risk of angina or a heart attack.

Apart from hypertension, other causes of heart failure include:

- CHD
- disease of heart muscle (cardiomyopathy)
- heart valve disease (aortic or mitral incompetence or stenosis)
- extra workload demands on the heart such as due to anaemia, overactive thyroid
- altered heart rhythm (arrhythmias).

IRREGULAR HEART BEAT

If high blood pressure puts the heart under enough strain or causes thickening and dilation of heart muscle, it may affect the way electricity is conducted through the heart. This can trigger abnormal heart rhythms (arrhythmias) such as atrial fibrillation, in which the two upper chambers of the heart beat out of synchronization with the ventricles – usually at a much faster rate. This produces an irregular, erratic pulse as the atria are not pumping blood into the ventricles in a co-ordinated fashion and cardiac output is affected.

CHD itself can also trigger arrhythmias due to lack of oxygen to the heart muscle so that it cannot conduct electricity properly, especially if this affects the part of the heart responsible for triggering the heart beat (the sinus node).

Chapter Six

HIGH BLOOD PRESSURE AND STROKE

High blood pressure is one of the main causes of stroke. In fact, those in their early forties with uncontrolled hypertension are 30 times more likely to have a stroke than those with normal blood pressure.

Stroke is a major cause of death and disability in the developed world. Each year it accounts for 1 death per 10,000 population in those aged 40, rising to 1 death per 100 aged 75. If people with hypertension had their blood pressure well controlled, the incidence of stroke would plummet.

WHAT IS A STROKE?

A stroke is a sudden loss of control of one or more body functions due to interruption of the blood supply to part of the brain, resulting in the death of some brain cells (neurones). High blood pressure is linked with several different types of stroke:

- a clot (thrombosis) in a brain artery which cuts off the supply of oxygen-rich blood to a variable number of brain cells so that they die (cerebral infarction)
- a clot that forms elsewhere in the circulation (such as in a carotid artery in the neck) which may break off and travel in the bloodstream (embolism) to the brain, where it becomes lodged in a blood vessel to cut off the blood supply suddenly
- haemorrhage into the brain due to a ruptured blood vessel.

Usually, the small arteries in the brain can dilate or constrict to adapt automatically to changes in BP, so that pressure remains relatively constant in the brain. As a result, blood flow to brain tissues can be maintained between systolic blood pressures of 80 and 170 mmHg. This autoregulation of blood flow in the brain can fail in severe hypertension when systolic blood pressure goes above 180 mmHg. As a result, blood pressure in cerebral arteries may suddenly rise. Haemorrhagic strokes may be linked with high blood pressure alone, as the greater the pressure, the more likely a blood vessel is to burst. Most types of stroke, however – haemorrhagic and clotting types – are linked with a combination of hypertension, atherosclerosis and increased stickiness of the blood.

Symptoms

The symptoms and signs produced by a stroke vary from person to person depending on the part of the brain affected and the number of brain cells that have died. The effects usually come on quickly and may get worse over a period of several hours. By definition, the symptoms last longer than 24 hours (if the victim survives). Typically, a stroke can produce one or more of the following:

- sudden loss of consciousness
- confusion or loss of memory
- loss of movement of part of the body (such as a limb) or several parts, usually on just one side of the body)
- loss of sensation in part of the body
- difficulty with speech
- difficulty swallowing
- double vision
- vomiting.

Transient Ischaemic Attacks

A transient ischaemic attack (TIA) is similar to a mini-stroke, in which symptoms get totally better within 24 hours. TIAs are often recurrent and are caused by small platelet clumps lodging in small blood vessels within the brain to block the circulation to some brain cells temporarily. The platelet clots break up and clear before brain cells die from lack of blood, however.

TIAs can occur in hypertensive patients when small platelet clots collect in damaged areas of the circulation between the heart and the head. The most common sites for clot formation are:

- the carotid arteries
- the vertebral arteries
- on a damaged heart valve
- in the left atrium when the upper chambers of the heart are beating out of synchronization with the ventricles (atrial fibrillation).

These clots may break up immediately after being formed, or may travel in the circulation to lodge in the brain, where they temporarily disrupt cerebral blood flow. TIAs can also occur due to a sudden fall in blood pressure (as can be caused by a heart arrhythmia).

A TIA is an important warning sign that a stroke may occur in the future – five years on from a TIA, 1 in 6 sufferers will have suffered a stroke, and 1 in 4 will have died, usually from a heart attack or stroke. If TIAs are treated by taking a drug that lowers platelet stickiness (such as aspirin), a full-blown stroke can often be prevented.

Sub-arachnoid Haemorrhage

A sub-arachnoid haemorrhage is bleeding into tissues surrounding the brain (sub-arachnoid space) due to rupture of a weakness in one of the arteries. This weakness is often congenital and due to a pouch-like widening of part of the artery wall (aneurysm). A sub-arachnoid haemorrhage causes sudden collapse and a violent headache which patients describe as feeling like a sudden, heavy blow to the back of the head. This is usually accompanied by vomiting, drowsiness or loss of consciousness.

Lacunar Infarctions

In some deceased patients who had hypertension, small areas of brain cell death (less than 1.5 cubic centimetres) are seen at post-mortem examination. These areas are known as lacunes and, depending on where they occur, may be symptomless or may produce symptoms such as a sudden loss of sensation (numbness) in a part of the body, a sudden difficulty in speaking or a clumsy hand, etc.

Dementia

If multiple areas of damage (lacunes) occur in the brain, a general decline in intellect usually occurs in people with atherosclerosis affecting the arterial system in the brain, especially if high blood pressure is also present. Multiple small strokes occur as a result of small clots forming, or of decreased blood supply through narrowed, furred up small arteries. The person affected usually deteriorates in a step-wise fashion with each subsequent small infarct. The end result is often dementia and difficulty in walking, resulting in a shuffling gait. This condition, multi-infarct dementia, used to be known as 'atherosclerotic parkinsonism'.

Recent research shows that someone with untreated raised blood pressure at the age of 70 is more likely to develop dementia within the next 15 years than a 70-year-old with normal BP – this applies to both the common forms of dementia, multi-infarct dementia and Alzheimer's disease. Alzheimer's disease is a form of dementia in which a widespread loss of brain cells is associated with the laying down of excess amounts of protein in the brain. Deposits of beta-amyloid protein form areas called plaques, while deposits of thread-like tau protein (which usually forms part of a cell's internal skeleton) form so-called tangles. Why Alzheimer's disease is linked with high blood pressure is not yet understood, but is probably due to increased risk of atherosclerosis and poor blood supply to the brain.

PREVENTING A STROKE

The single most important factor in preventing a stroke is to bring your high blood pressure under control. If blood pressure has been high for a long time, this may have to be done slowly, as suddenly lowering the pressure down to normal may affect blood flow to parts of the brain where circulation is poor. Other risk factors that need to be addressed are similar to those linked with coronary heart disease:

- stop smoking
- lose any excess weight
- exercise regularly
- keep alcohol intake within the recommended safe amounts
- take steps to lower raised blood fat levels
- if you have diabetes, make sure your blood sugar levels are always well controlled
- if you are prone to high blood pressure, avoid any drugs that may put blood pressure up
- new research confirms that people with the highest intakes of vitamin C are half as likely to suffer a stroke as those with intakes of less than 28 mg vitamin C per day
- a review of 25 studies shows that taking low dose aspirin (75–150 mg) per day can reduce the risk of a heart attack or stroke by 30 per cent, and the risk of dying from either by 15 per cent (*see Chapter 8*).

Homocysteine

If you have hypertension, your risk of a stroke is more likely if you have raised blood levels of the amino acid, homocysteine (*see page 30*).

Chapter Seven

OTHER COMPLICATIONS

As well as triggering atherosclerosis, coronary heart disease and stroke, uncontrolled hypertension is associated with other potentially serious problems, including:

- kidney damage
- damage to the back of the eye (retina)
- aortic aneurysm
- peripheral vascular disease with poor circulation to the peripheries (such as the limbs).

Blood vessel walls subjected to long-term untreated hypertension show several changes. They become tortuous, thickened and furred up. If blood pressure is very high (such as in malignant hypertension, *see page 31*), the vessel walls may start to crumble. This process is known as fibrinoid necrosis. The damaged vessel walls start to leak so that protein-rich fluid or even whole blood seeps out of the bloodstream into surrounding tissues. As well as interfering with blood supply to that part of the body, the leakages cause damage, inflammation and scarring. This is referred to as target organ damage.

KIDNEY DAMAGE

High blood pressure can be the cause or the result of renal disease, and it can be difficult to tell the two apart.

When it is the cause, benign essential hypertension leads to hardening and furring up of the large renal arteries and also damages small blood vessels in the kidney:

- the walls of small vessels thicken and the lining takes on a glassy appearance (hyalinization)
- in larger vessels, the inner part of the wall doubles up and the lining proliferates to form concentric thickenings that give an onion-skin appearance.

These changes occur in vessels taking blood to kidney tissues, so the kidneys may start to shrink (atrophy) due to poor blood supply. At the same time, poor blood supply to the kidney filtering units (nephrons) means that less urine is produced and kidney function progressively deteriorates. Damage due to high blood pressure also makes the small blood vessels leaky, so that protein is found in the urine (proteinuria). This is an important early sign of many kidney diseases and the reason you should ideally have your urine checked regularly for protein when visiting your doctor's surgery.

If left untreated, high blood pressure would eventually lead to kidney failure, in which fluid and salts build up in the body. Fortunately, most patients with hypertension can be protected against kidney failure by having their blood pressure well controlled with drugs. Kidney failure is still sometimes seen where blood pressure and diabetes occur together, as there are then two disease processes causing kidney damage and this is less easy to control totally.

Poor blood supply to the kidneys in turn stimulates the baroreceptor pressure monitors in the kidneys. This triggers increased production of renin hormone, leading to activation of the renin-angiotensin system (*see page 15*). This quickly puts blood pressure up in the body's attempt to increase the blood supply to the kidneys. This puts your blood pressure up even more, so a vicious cycle is set in place.

Similarly, kidney diseases (such as those due to inflammation of the kidney tubules) can put blood pressure up and cause hypertension in the first place. This is because poor kidney function results in the build-up of fluid and salts in the body, leading to a rise in BP and secondary hypertension. Narrowing of a renal artery leading to one kidney will mean that blood reaches that kidney under low pressure. This in turn activates the renin-angiotensin system, again leading to secondary hypertension.

If blood tests show that your levels of kidney chemicals (urea and creatinine) are abnormal, you will need further tests to assess renal function. These include:

- additional blood tests to see how well your kidneys are filtering your blood (creatinine clearance rate)
- an intravenous urogram – a substance that shows up on x-ray is injected into your bloodstream and a series of x-rays taken to show how well your kidneys concentrate the dye. This also outlines your urinary system and shows up any anatomical abnormalities or shrinkage of the kidneys.
- ultrasound of your kidneys.

EYE DAMAGE

High blood pressure damages small arteries throughout your body. Those in the back of the eye have the advantage of being visible using an ophthalmoscope, and show the state of arterioles throughout your bodily systems – including your brain. Early changes due to hypertension include thickening of retinal blood vessel walls. If hypertension becomes long-standing or severe, the blood vessels leak and little haemorrhages form. Other changes are probably due to obstruction of vessels and reduced blood circulation.

If your blood pressure has been high, your doctor will regularly check the back of your eyes for signs of damage. This is performed in a darkened room using an instrument called an ophthalmoscope, which contains a number of lenses and a light source. Sometimes you may have one eye dilated first with drops to make the task easier. The doctor is looking for various abnormalities known as Keith-Wagener retinal changes. These are divided into four stages of severity:

Grade 1   increased tortuosity of retinal arteries which, because they are thickened and bulging under pressure, also reflect light from the ophthalmoscope more than usual. This gives them an appearance known as silver wiring.

Grade 2   as in Grade 1, plus evidence that the thickened, bulging arteries are compressing the veins where they cross over them (arterio-venous nipping)

Grade 3   as in Grade 2, plus signs that the arteries have started leaking – leakage of protein-rich fluid produces white, soft, 'cotton-wool' like exudates, while leakage of blood produces flame-shaped haemorrhages

Grade 4   as in Grade 3, plus swelling, bulging and blurring of the head of the optic nerve (papilloedema).

If haemorrhages, exudates or papilloedema are visible in the back of the eye, it shows that malignant hypertension has developed. These are the same sort of processes that are occurring in the brain and which are thought to lead to a stroke. It is very important that your hypertension is brought under control quickly and safely. You may be admitted to hospital for complete bed rest while your drug treatment is adjusted.

AORTIC ANEURYSM

The walls of the largest artery in your body – the aorta – are under a lot of pressure. If they become hardened and furred up, the pressure may cause the aorta to dilate. This produces a bulge known as an aneurysm, usually in the abdomen (although they can occur in the chest). The aneurysm may slowly increase in size and cause severe stretch pains (that is, pain caused by stretching of the aorta). If the aneurysm expands to a diameter greater than 6 cm it may eventually burst (ruptured aortic aneurysm). This is a potentially fatal surgical emergency needing rapid repair with a graft. The aneurysm can also split lengthways if blood seeps into its wall (dissecting aortic aneurysm).

Where possible, aortic aneurysms are replaced in a planned procedure before they have threatened to rupture.

PERIPHERAL VASCULAR DISEASE

Hardening and furring up of the arteries throughout your body can lead to peripheral vascular disease, in which blood supply to your legs is severely limited. Even a mild increase in exercise means that your muscles need extra blood and oxygen – if these cannot be supplied, your leg muscles will start to cramp. This causes a severe pain in the calf muscles which comes on during exercise and stops when you rest – a condition called intermittent claudication. If your blood supply is severely affected, even walking 100 metres or less on the flat can bring symptoms on. If blood supply is very poor, ischaemic pain may occur at rest, tissues may break down to form a leg ulcer and eventually gangrene may set in. Severe peripheral vascular disease is most likely in someone with hypertension who also smokes, and/or who also suffers from diabetes.

Aspirin will help to thin the blood and improve blood supply. Some tablets also work by increasing the flexibility of red blood cells so they can squeeze through small blood vessels more easily. Interestingly, research shows that taking garlic powder tablets can improve peripheral circulation enough to increase the distance you can walk before calf pain starts by up to 30 per cent in three months.

A severely narrowed artery in the leg can be overcome with a by-pass graft to open up an alternative circulatory route. If there are only one or two main sites of blockage, these can sometimes be overcome by passing a balloon catheter into the artery and expanding it at the site of the blockage to dilate the vessel locally.

Impotence

Peripheral vascular disease can cause sexual difficulties in men. Poor blood supply to the penis results in problems with achieving or maintaining an erection. Impotence is a common and distressing condition affecting 10 to 30 per cent of men on a regular basis. Unfortunately, due to embarrassment or a mistaken belief that nothing can be done, victims often suffer in silence and despair. In 9 out of 10 cases, impotence can be corrected.

If you wake with an erection in the morning, then there is probably little physically wrong. You may be overtired and stressed or be suffering from drug side-effects. If you don't wake with an erection, you may again be suffering from drug side-effects, but you could also have hardening and furring up of the arteries supplying blood to the penis, or excessively leaky veins which are allowing blood to drain back out of your penis too quickly.

The treatment of impotence is now sophisticated:

- Male hormone replacement therapy or treatment to lower certain hormone levels may work if your problem is hormonal.
- The penis can be placed in a cylinder from which the air is extracted. This causes the penis to inflate. A tight ring is then placed around the base of the shaft to trap blood so the penis remains erect when the vacuum cylinder is removed. (Obviously this ring can only be left in place for a short while.)
- You can be taught to give injections into the shaft of your penis. This is known as PIPE, which stands for Pharmacologically Induced Penile Erections, and is said to be no more painful than a mosquito bite.
- New drug treatments are becoming available in the form of a topical gel or cream which you rub onto the penis.
- Surgery can be performed to declog or by-pass furred-up arteries, or tighten leaking veins.
- A prosthesis can be implanted. These are of two main types:
  1. semi-rigid rods which give you half an erection all of the time
  2. inflatable devices with a small pump implanted in the scrotum and a reservoir of fluid in a bag in the abdomen. These are activated by a trigger button on the scrotal pump.
- If the problem is psychological, counselling and psychotherapy can help.

If you do develop impotence, do pluck up courage to see your doctor. In many cases, a change in your anti-hypertensive medication is all that is needed. If the problem is more complex, referral to a specialist (urologist) will usually find the cause and offer a cure.

Chapter Eight

DRUG TREATMENTS FOR HIGH BLOOD PRESSURE

Doctors are given guidelines that help them to decide which patients with high blood pressure need treatment and which don't. Basically, if your BP is consistently found to be above a certain level, it is important to bring it down to normal levels to reduce your risk of future complications such as coronary heart disease (CHD), kidney failure, eye problems (hypertensive retinopathy) or stroke. If complications (target organ damage) are already in evidence, your management will be stepped up.

These guidelines are based on extensive outcome studies and trials that confirm the health benefits of treatment. In some cases, the blood pressure may be borderline and research may not show clear benefits of treatment. In this case, your doctor will monitor you regularly to make sure your BP does not go up further. Diet and lifestyle changes may be enough to help to control your BP so that you don't need to take drug treatment (*see Chapter 10*).

Before deciding to start treatment, the doctor needs to be sure that your high blood pressure is consistent. You will therefore have your BP measured several times on different occasions to see if it comes down. If your BP seems high at the start of a consultation, you will have it rechecked at the end of your appointment when it may well have come down significantly. This short-term risk in BP is linked with the stress and adrenaline surge of visiting the surgery. In some people, the effect is so pronounced that the BP can surge upwards by 30 mmHg or more – systolic rises as high as 100 mmHg have been recorded. This is known as White Coat Hypertension. If this condition is suspected, your blood pressure will be monitored continuously over a 24-hour period by a small electronic recording device attached to a belt you wear around your waist. You may also be taught how to measure your own blood pressure at home.

Blood pressure rises with age, and studies have shown that taking steps to lower high BP is beneficial to health. Until recently, the benefits of drug treatment in the elderly were less clear cut, but new research shows that controlling hypertension with drugs:

- lowers the risk of stroke by 35 per cent
- reduces the risk of heart complications by 20 per cent
- reduces overall risk of death at any age by 15 per cent.

Treatment of hypertension in the elderly should therefore be started over a threshold BP of 160/90.

The aim of treatment is to lower your blood pressure gradually over a period of time. Your doctor will start you off on a low dose of tablets to see how your blood pressure responds. If this is not enough, your dose may be increased, other drugs may be added in, or your medication may be completely changed. In some cases, more than one drug may be needed to achieve an acceptable BP. It may seem annoying to have to take one, two or even three different kinds of drugs when you feel perfectly well, but by prescribing treatment to keep your blood pressure within normal limits your doctor is helping you to avoid the complications of uncontrolled hypertension – heart attack, stroke, peripheral vascular disease, kidney failure and even blindness.

It is important to take your blood pressure tablets regularly as prescribed. Some tablets need only be taken once a day, but others may need to be taken two or more times daily. This depends on how long each dose of medicine works in your body, and on how bad your blood pressure is.

When most forms of anti-hypertensive treatments are stopped, blood pressure only climbs up slowly over several days or even weeks. With some forms of treatment, however, a rebound effect can occur rapidly, making your blood pressure shoot back up.

Don't stop taking any blood pressure treatment without first consulting your doctor. If you notice something that may be a side-effect, such as a rash, dizziness or sexual problems, always tell your doctor straightaway so your dose can be altered or your treatment changed to one that suits you better.

IF YOU SHOULD FORGET TO TAKE YOUR MEDICATION

If you do forget to take your treatment occasionally, it is unlikely that you will come to any harm. If you forget your tablets on a regular basis, you may run into problems.

- If your treatment is only a few hours late, take it as soon as you remember.
- If you have missed one dose and your next one is already due, just take one dose – DON'T take two at once. Be especially careful not to miss any further doses.
- If you forget to take your blood pressure treatment for more than one or two days, contact your doctor for further advice.

TIPS TO HELP YOU REMEMBER TO TAKE YOUR MEDICATION

- Try to take your blood pressure treatment regularly, at the same time every day so you get into a routine.
- Write a note for yourself and stick it up somewhere that you will easily see it.
- Keep your tablets/capsules somewhere that you can remember them easily – such as with your toothpaste (but make sure they are out of the reach of children).
- Keep your tablets in a special dispenser box marked with separate containers for different times of the day.
- If you have a programmable alarm watch, set it for when your medicine is due.
- If you live with someone else, ask them to help you remember.
- Make sure you get your next prescription in plenty of time so you don't run out.
- If you are going away, take enough tablets with you to last the whole time.

TYPICAL GUIDELINES FOR DOCTORS TREATING HYPERTENSION

Measurement: baseline BP established by taking 2–3 BP readings per visit (while patient is seated) on up to 4 occasions

Aims of Treatment: to reduce diastolic BP to less than 90 mmHg
to reduce systolic BP to less than 160 mmHg

Risk Factors: complications (target organ damage); being male; being a smoker; age; BP towards upper limit of range; family history of cardio-vascular disease; having diabetes; high blood fat (lipid) levels

Complications (Target Organ Damage): Left ventricle of heart enlarged (hypertrophy); angina; transient ischaemia attacks (TIAs); stroke; peripheral vascular disease; heart attack; kidney function impaired.

DIASTOLIC BP	COMPLICATIONS	RECOMMENDED ACTION
90–99 mmHg	None	Start diet and lifestyle changes immediately. BP monitored for several months. If BP does not respond, drug treatment started if patient is over 60 or has several other risk factors for CHD.
90–99 mmHg	Present	Measure BP repeatedly over 3–6 months. Start diet and lifestyle changes immediately. Start drug treatment after 6 months if BP does not respond.
100–109 mmHg	None	Measure BP on 3 or more occasions over a week or so. Start diet and lifestyle changes immediately. If BP drops below 100 mmHg, continue monitoring. If BP stays at 100 mmHg or above, start drug treatment.
100–109 mmHg	Present	Measure BP on 3 or more occasions over a week or so, then monthly. Start diet and lifestyle changes immediately. Start drug treatment if BP remains high.
110 mmHg	+/–	Measure BP repeatedly over 1–2 weeks. Start diet and lifestyle changes immediately. Start drug treatment immediately if BP stays high.

DIASTOLIC BP	COMPLICATIONS	RECOMMENDED ACTION
160 mmHg	None	Measure BP repeatedly over 1 – 2 weeks. Start diet and lifestyle changes immediately.
		If systolic 160–190 mmHg and diastolic less than 95 mmHg, monitor for 3–6 months. Start drug treatment if systolic remains greater than 160 mmHg.
		If systolic is 200 mmHg or above, or if systolic is 160–190 mmHg and diastolic 95 mmHg or above, start drug treatment immediately.
More than 160 mmHg	Present	Start drug treatment immediately. Start diet and lifestyle changes immediately.

Diet and Lifestyle changes: Lose any excess weight; stop smoking; reduce salt intake; reduce dietary fat intake; reduce stress levels; take more exercise; limit weekly alcohol intake to less than 21 units (men), less than 14 units (women), plus have alcohol-free days.

Treatment: Diuretics, beta-blockers, ACE inhibitors, calcium antagonists, alpha-antagonists. Consider lipid-lowering drugs if blood fat levels are raised.

Follow-up: Measure BP frequently; ensure diastolic BP is maintained between 80–90 mmHg with 3-monthly monitoring; step down treatment if diastolic BP remains below 80 mmHg; continue diet and lifestyle changes.

Refer: Patients with malignant (accelerated) or refractory hypertension should be referred to a specialist.

DRUG TREATMENT

At present, five classes of drug are used as first-line treatments to lower high blood pressure. Each doctor has to decide which drug to use for a particular patient. There are two schools of thought:

1. Traditionalists prefer to use older drugs – diuretics and beta-blockers – which have been tried and tested for 30 years or more. These lower blood pressure, protect against strokes and, in the elderly, protect against heart attacks as well. They can cause a number of side-effects, however (such as dizziness, tiredness, impotence) that can affect the quality of life in some patients.
2. Modernists prefer to use the newer classes of drugs which have only been around for 15 years – calcium channel antagonists, ACE inhibitors, alpha-antagonists – which are just as effective at lowering blood pressure. Results from large, long-term studies to show how well these treatments protect against heart attack or stroke are not always available, however, although short-term studies suggest they are beneficial. These drugs tend to have fewer contraindications and fewer side-effects in some patients such as those with hypertension and diabetes, or those with hypertension and heart failure.

In general, doctors are moving towards tailoring drug treatment to suit an individual patient's needs rather than following a blanket approach. Drugs are started at the lowest dose and slowly raised as necessary if BP does not respond.

Is Anti-hypertensive Treatment for Life?

Once drug treatment is started for high blood pressure, it is often for life. However, if you don't have any complications from your high blood pressure and you have managed to make diet and lifestyle changes that naturally bring your blood pressure down, it may be possible to reduce your tablet dose or to withdraw it altogether. You should never alter your medication or stop it suddenly yourself, however. If your doctor decides to withdraw your treatment this is usually done slowly in a stepwise fashion to prevent sudden rebound hypertension. You will be followed up closely over a long period of time, as in some cases BP starts to creep back up again after six months, a year or more.

How Successful Is Blood Pressure Treatment?

According to experts, if you ask most doctors they will say that 80 per cent of their patients with high blood pressure have their condition well controlled. In reality, however, research shows that 50 to 60 per cent of patients with high blood pressure are actually poorly controlled. This is as true in hospital clinics as it is in general practice.

When told this, doctors tend to blame their patients for not taking their tablets as prescribed. While this is sometimes true, the main reason seems to be that once a doctor has started a patient on treatment, the doctor doesn't alter the dose or change the treatment if the patient's blood pressure doesn't respond. In one study, 60 per cent of patients had never had their medications changed, or the dose altered since it was first prescribed.

You therefore need to take a close interest in your own blood pressure and how well it is controlled. If it seems to be staying high, try suggesting to your doctor that your drug treatment may need review. Similarly, if your BP drops nicely as a result of losing excess weight, taking more exercise, stopping smoking, avoiding alcohol and cutting back on salt and caffeine, try asking your doctor if your drug dose might be lowered – or even slowly withdrawn altogether. If changes are made to your treatment, don't forget that you will need to attend surgery regularly to have your BP closely monitored until it has stabilized. Although this may seem a pain – especially as you probably have no symptoms to complain of – it is vitally important for your future health. Your dedication will also encourage the co-operation of your doctor in individually fine-tuning your blood pressure treatment.

DRUGS USED TO TREAT HIGH BLOOD PRESSURE

The aim of treatment is to reduce diastolic BP to below 90 mmHg and/or reduce systolic BP to below 160 mmHg.

Five main groups of drugs are used: diuretics, beta-blockers, alpha-blockers, calcium channel blockers, and ACE inhibitors.

Diuretics (Water Tablets)

The types of diuretics used to treat high blood pressure are the thiazide diuretics such as bendrofluazide, cyclopenthiazide, hydrochlorothiazide, hydroflumethiazide, polythiazide. In general, diuretics are used as a first-line treatment in the elderly, or are combined with other anti-hypertensive drugs (such as a beta-blocker or ACE inhibitor) to boost its action in younger patients.

They lower blood pressure by increasing loss of salts through the kidney into the urine. This tends to draw fluid out of the circulation, causes mild dilation of small arteries and lowers arteriolar resistance. The diuretics act within 1–2 hours of being given and are usually taken in the morning so you do not have to get up at night to pass water. When you first start taking the tablets, you may notice that you have to pass water more frequently than usual for the first few days, then this effect tends to disappear as dilation of the arterioles occurs. Only low doses of thiazide diuretic are needed to bring your diastolic BP down by around 5 mmHg – higher doses have no further effect on BP and are more likely to cause side-effects.

Thiazide diuretics are usually well tolerated in the low doses used, but possible side-effects due to the way they affect your metabolism can occur at higher doses.

POSSIBLE SIDE-EFFECTS

- low potassium levels – monitoring of blood electrolytes will help to detect this; it is usually treated by adding in another sort of diuretic that conserves body potassium levels, rather than by giving potassium supplements
- raised blood sugar levels – thiazide diuretics should not be used in people with diabetes, as they can affect blood sugar control
- raised uric acid levels leading to gout
- raised blood calcium levels
- raised blood fat levels
- impotence
- rashes – including those due to light-sensitivity

- feelings of tiredness all the time
- feeling faint on standing up (postural hypotension)
- mild nausea or other gut upsets.

Thiazides are only used with caution and close monitoring in the elderly, when given to pregnant or breastfeeding women, and in people with systemic lupus erythematosus (SLE) or with kidney or liver problems.

They should not be used in people with diabetes, sodium/ potassium/calcium imbalances, severe kidney or liver problems, active gout or Addison's disease.

Beta-blockers

The beta-blockers are used to treat both high blood pressure and angina. There are two sorts of beta receptors in the body and different drugs block these to different extents:

β-1 blockers	interfere with receptors in the heart
β-2 blockers	interfere with receptors in the peripheral blood vessels, lung airways (bronchi), pancreas, kidneys and liver.

The way β-blockers lower blood pressure is not fully understood, but they are thought to:

- damp down nerve pathways to interfere with blood vessel constriction
- slow the heart rate to around 60 beats per minute
- reduce the force of contraction of the heart
- decrease the workload of the heart and cardiac output
- lower secretion of a kidney hormone, renin (*see page 15*)
- reduce sensitivity of blood pressure sensors (baroreceptors)
- block stress hormone (adrenaline) receptors
- have some action on the brain.

In general, beta-blockers are used as a first-line treatment in young people with hypertension and in patients who have CHD. Because they also affect receptors in the lungs, they should not be used in patients with asthma as they can trigger an asthma attack. They should also be avoided in people with heart failure as they may reduce heart activity so much that they trigger more serious heart pump failure. β-blockers may be less effective in people of Afro-Caribbean descent unless combined with a thiazide diuretic.

Beta-blockers have been shown to reduce significantly the risk of having a second heart attack and may prolong life in high-risk individuals.

POSSIBLE SIDE-EFFECTS

- reduced circulation to the peripheries, leading to cold extremities
- Raynaud's phenomenon due to constriction of arteries in the digits (fingers/toes go white and numb through poor blood supply)
- impotence
- fatigue
- adverse changes in blood fat (lipid) levels
- constriction of airways (bronchospasm)
- exacerbation of congestive heart pump failure
- reduced tolerance for exercise
- sleep disturbances, including nightmares
- slight deterioration in sugar control in people with diabetes
- dry eyes
- skin rash
- mild nausea or other gut upsets.

Beta-blockers should not be withdrawn suddenly, but must be tailed off slowly so that rebound high blood pressure (or angina) does not occur.

The older, first-generation β-blockers (such as propranolol, oxprenolol) are non-selective in that they block both β-1 and β-2 receptors.

Second-generation β-blockers (such as atenolol, bisoprolol, metoprolol) are more selective and mainly block receptors in the heart rather than those elsewhere in the body, so are less likely to produce some unwanted side-effects such as triggering an asthma attack or lowering HDL-cholesterol.

The new third-generation β-blockers (such as celiprolol) also help to dilate peripheral blood vessels, which helps to reduce side-effects of poor blood supply to the peripheries and changes in blood fat levels.

Some drugs also affect other receptors, known as alpha-receptors (see below) – so they have both β-blocking and α-blocking actions (such as carvedilol, labetalol). This helps to reduce side-effects of poor blood supply to the peripheries and changes in blood fat levels.

β-blockers should not be taken by people with:

- some heart rhythm problems (second- or third-degree AV block; sinus bradycardia, sick sinus syndrome)
- severe peripheral vascular disease (a result of long-term high blood pressure and atherosclerosis, *see page 43*)
- congestive cardiac failure (*see page 49*)
- low blood pressure
- untreated phaeochromocytoma (a type of tumour, usually of the adrenal glands) which causes one type of secondary hypertension
- asthma or obstructive airways disease (unless a cardioselective β-1 blocker is tried with caution if there are compelling reasons).

They should only be used with caution and close monitoring in people with diabetes, metabolic acidosis, liver or kidney problems or an overactive thyroid, or in women who are pregnant or breastfeeding.

Alpha-blockers

Alpha-blockers (such as doxazosin, indoramin, prazosin, terazosin) lower blood pressure by dilating both arteries and veins. They sometimes cause a rapid fall in blood pressure after the first dose and treatment should be started with caution – usually at night so that if low blood pressure does occur, this is after you have retired to bed. Indoramin has more side-effects than the other α-blockers and, if taking it, you should avoid alcohol as this drug boosts alcohol absorption.

POSSIBLE SIDE-EFFECTS

- dizziness on standing up due to low blood pressure
- headache
- fatigue
- weakness
- stuffy nose (rhinitis)
- dry mouth
- fluid retention with swelling of tissues (oedema)
- sleepiness
- nausea
- weight gain
- palpitations
- urinary incontinence has been reported
- failure of ejaculation has been reported.

Calcium Channel Blockers

Calcium channel blockers (such as amlodipine, diltiazem, felodipine, isradipine, lacidipine, nicardipine, nifedipine, verapamil) are used to treat both high blood pressure and angina. They work by:

- blocking the transport of calcium ions through cell membranes
- relaxing muscles in arterial walls and reducing arterial spasm
- dilating peripheral veins to encourage pooling of blood
- reducing the force of contraction of the heart.

POSSIBLE SIDE-EFFECTS

- facial flushing
- headache
- fatigue
- nausea
- swollen gums
- swollen ankles
- constipation
- skin rashes
- weight gain

- abdominal discomfort
- palpitations or heart arrhythmias with some calcium channel blockers.

Calcium channel blockers should not be used in patients who:

- have heart failure
- have certain heart rhythm problems (severe bradycardia, second- or third-degree AV block; sick sinus syndrome – unless a pacemaker is fitted)
- suffer from advanced aortic stenosis
- have porphyria (a metabolic disease)
- are pregnant.

Treatment must not be stopped suddenly, but should be tailed off slowly to prevent rebound angina. Verapamil is slightly different from the others in the way it works, and should not be used together with a β-blocker.

ACE Inhibitors

ACE inhibitor drugs are so-named because they block formation of Angiotensin Converting Enzyme (ACE). This prevents formation of angiotensin II (*see Chapter 2*) – a powerful constrictor of blood vessels, leading to dilation of both arterioles and veins. This reduces total peripheral resistance and arterial blood pressure. ACE inhibitors also suppress the production of aldosterone (*see page 17*) and increase blood flow to the kidneys, so more fluid and sodium are lost as urine. They are usually considered for treating hypertension when thiazides or betablockers are contraindicated, not tolerated, or fail to control high blood pressure.

They can cause a sudden fall in BP on giving the first dose, especially in patients who are taking diuretics or who are dehydrated. Where possible, diuretic treatment is therefore usually stopped a few days before ACE inhibitor treatment is started. For some, the first dose is best taken at night on retiring to bed. Kidney function and salt balance should be checked before treatment is started.

ACE inhibitors may be less effective in people of Afro-Caribbean descent unless combined with a thiazide diuretic.

POSSIBLE SIDE-EFFECTS

- chronic, dry cough
- voice changes
- dizziness
- taste disturbances
- fluid retention (oedema)
- fatigue
- nausea
- indigestion
- abdominal discomfort
- diarrhoea
- constipation
- high blood potassium levels
- muscle cramps
- tissue swelling
- rashes
- sleep disturbances
- blood disorders
- impotence
- hair loss
- mood changes.

ACE inhibitors should not be taken:

- in pregnancy
- by patients with renal blood vessel disease (stenosis)
- by those with aortic stenosis
- by patients suffering porphyria.

ANGIOTENSIN II ANTAGONISTS

This is a new class of drug that has only recently become available (such as losartan). It is similar to the ACE inhibitors except that instead of inhibiting angiotensin converting enzyme, it blocks angiotensin II to produce similar effects. It dilates blood vessels, stimulates kidney function and may also have a direct action on the brain to reduce drinking and increase urine output. At present, it is mainly used in people who develop a persistent dry cough as a troublesome side-effect of the ACE inhibitors, as it does not produce this problem.

Other Drugs

Occasionally, drugs from the above groups may not be sufficient or suitable for treating an individual case of high blood pressure. Two other drugs may occasionally be used: hydralazine or methyldopa.

HYDRALAZINE

This vasodilator lowers blood pressure by relaxing arteries and increasing their diameter. When used to treat hypertension, it is usually combined with a beta-blocker and thiazide diuretic to stop the heart rate and cardiac output from increasing and to avoid fluid retention. It may cause a very rapid drop in blood pressure.

POSSIBLE SIDE-EFFECTS

- nausea and vomiting
- flushing
- headache
- rapid pulse rate
- fluid retention (oedema)
- angina
- an immune problem resembling systemic lupus erythematosus (SLE) with weight loss, joint pains, muscle aches and non-specific symptoms of being unwell
- rash
- fever
- liver or kidney problems
- paralytic ileus (inactivity of the bowel)
- peripheral neuritis (nerve inflammation)
- some blood disorders.

Hydralazine should not be taken by people with:

- SLE
- porphyria
- very rapid heart beat
- heart failure
- some types of heart problem related to obstruction of blood flow.

It should only be used with caution in people with CHD, kidney problems, cerebro-vascular disease and during pregnancy or when breastfeeding.

Methyldopa

This used to be the most popular drug for treating high blood pressure, and may still be taken by elderly patients started on it many years ago. It lowers blood pressure by acting on the brain to trigger nerve actions that reduce heart output, urine production and arteriolar constriction. Methyldopa is often used together with a diuretic. It is particularly useful for controlling high blood pressure in pregnancy. It may cause a rapid fall in blood pressure, especially in the elderly.

POSSIBLE SIDE-EFFECTS

- dry mouth
- drowsiness
- sedation
- depression
- diarrhoea
- fluid retention
- difficulty with ejaculation
- liver problems
- anaemia
- an immune problem resembling systemic lupus erythematosus (SLE)
- parkinsonism
- rashes
- nasal stuffiness

Methyldopa should not be taken by people with:

- a history of depression
- active liver disease
- porphyria
- phaeochromocytoma (a tumour of the adrenal glands or nervous system).

DRUGS USED TO LOWER HIGH BLOOD CHOLESTEROL LEVELS

The blood pressure treatment guidelines suggest that lipid-lowering drugs should be considered if blood fat levels are raised.

The best way to reduce high cholesterol levels is through dietary changes (low-fat diet, using olive oil, rapeseed oil for cooking, eating oily fish, taking fish oil supplements, taking garlic powder tablets) and increasing exercise levels.

If total blood cholesterol is above 7.8 mmol/l and is mainly in the form of harmful LDL-cholesterol, a lipid-lowering drug may be prescribed if dietary changes have failed.

In some cases, raised cholesterol levels are due to hereditary difficulties with fat metabolism. In these cases, one or more drugs often have to be prescribed.

Resins

Resins (such as cholestyramine, colestipol) work by binding to bile acids and preventing their reabsorption in the gut. This interferes with regulatory messages feeding back to the liver, so that more cholesterol is broken down into bile acids and excreted from the body. They can lower LDL-cholesterol levels by up to 25 per cent on top of that achieved through dietary changes. Unfortunately, they cause triglycerides to rise by up to 5 per cent. They are mainly used when a statin cannot be taken (*see below*). Side-effects include constipation, lack of the fat-soluble vitamins A, D and K in long-term therapy.

Fibrates

Fibrates (such as bezafibrate, ciprofibrate, clofibrate, fenofibrate, gemfibrozil) work by lowering liver synthesis of cholesterol. They reduce total cholesterol by up to 25 per cent and triglycerides by up to 50 per cent. They also have a beneficial effect on types of cholesterol in the blood, raising HDL- and lowering LDL-cholesterol. Unfortunately, they can trigger muscle pain (myositis), especially in patients with kidney disease. Some encourage gallstones and inflammation of the gall bladder by increasing excretion of cholesterol into the bile. Other possible side-effects include fatigue, muscle cramps, dizziness, painful extremities, hair loss, blurred vision, impotence and, rarely, inability to feel sexual pleasure.

Statins

Statins (such as fluvastatin, pravastatin, simvastatin) work by inhibiting a liver enzyme and lowering cholesterol production in the liver. LDL-cholesterol can be reduced by up to 40 per cent, with a beneficial rise in HDL-cholesterol and a moderate reduction in triglycerides. Side-effects include reversible muscle problems, non-cardiac chest pain, diarrhoea, constipation, sinusitis, insomnia, flatulence and fatigue.

Nicotinic Acid Derivatives

These drugs (such as acipimox, nicofuranose, nicotinic acid) lower both triglycerides and cholesterol levels by inhibiting breakdown of body fat stores and inhibiting the production of fats in the liver. LDL-cholesterol can be lowered by up to 20 per cent, and HDL-cholesterol is increased. They are limited by their side-effects of blood vessel dilation causing dizziness, headache and flushing.

Marine Fish Oils

Marine omega-3 triglycerides are a natural product that reduce blood levels of cholesterol and harmful triglycerides by inhibiting their production in the liver. They make the blood less sticky and reduce the risk of arterial thrombosis. They have few side-effects apart from possible nausea (if too much is taken) and belching.

Probucal

This drug is in a class of its own whose precise mode of action is unknown. It seems to increase excretion of bile acids in the faeces, so that more cholesterol is broken down in the liver to replenish them. It can lower LDL-cholesterol by up to 10 per cent, but HDL-cholesterol is reduced as well. Triglycerides remain unchanged. Probucal also acts as an antioxidant. Possible side-effects include flatulence, diarrhoea, mild abdominal pain and, very rarely, abnormal heart rhythm.

Aspirin

Aspirin is a commonly used painkiller and anti-inflammatory drug that also has a powerful blood-thinning effect. It lowers the stickiness of platelet particles in the blood so that they are less likely to clump together and form unwanted clots. This effect occurs at only a quarter of the dose needed to relieve pain. Although there is not yet felt to be enough evidence to recommend that everyone takes prophylactic aspirin, people who should consider taking a mini-dose of aspirin regularly every day include those who have:

- angina
- suffered a previous heart attack
- had a coronary artery by-pass graft or dilation (angioplasty)
- had surgery for poor circulation in the limbs
- diabetes
- several major risk factors for CHD.

A review of 25 studies shows that taking low-dose aspirin (75 mg–150 mg) per day can reduce the risk of a heart attack or stroke by 30 per cent, and the risk of dying from either by 15 per cent.

If you fall into any of the above groups and are not taking a junior aspirin per day, check with your doctor that it will suit you and fit in with any other medication that you are taking.

Chapter Nine

COMPLEMENTARY THERAPIES

Some complementary treatments are helpful in bringing high blood pressure down. If your BP is borderline and you are not yet on any drug treatment, these therapies – combined with dietary and lifestyle changes – may be sufficient to stop you needing conventional drug treatment in the future. If you are already on anti-hypertensive medication, however, it is important to continue taking your drugs alongside any complementary treatments you decide to try. You should never stop taking a prescribed blood pressure lowering drug without your doctor's knowledge and consent – in some cases, withdrawing treatment rapidly can make your BP rebound up to a higher level than before you started treatment, putting your health at risk.

If consulting an alternative practitioner, bear in mind that standards of training and experience vary widely. Where possible:

- Select a therapist on the basis of personal recommendation from a satisfied client whom you know and whose opinion you trust.
- Check what qualifications the therapist has, and check his or her standing with the relevant umbrella organization for that therapy. The organization will be able to tell you what training their members have undertaken and their code of ethics, and can refer you to qualified practitioners in your area.
- Find out how long your course of treatment will last and how much it is likely to cost.
- Ask how much experience the practitioner has had in treating high blood pressure, and about his or her rate of success.

The following complementary therapies have helped many hypertensives, although just as with orthodox medicine, not every treatment will suit every individual.

ACUPUNCTURE

Acupuncture is based on the belief that life energy (*chi* or *qi*) flows through the body along 12 different channels called meridians. When this energy flow becomes blocked, symptoms of illness are triggered. By inserting fine needles into specific acupuncture points overlying these meridians, blockages are overcome and the flow of *qi* corrected or altered to relieve symptoms. Altogether, there are 365 acupoints in the body; your therapist will select which points to use depending on your individual symptoms. Fine, disposable needles are used, which cause little if any discomfort. You may notice a slight pricking sensation, or an odd tingling buzz as the needle is inserted a few millimetres into the skin. The needles are usually left in place for up to 20 minutes, and may be twiddled periodically. Sometimes a small cone of dried herbs is ignited and burned near the active acupoint to warm the skin. This is known as moxibustion. The best known effect of *qi* manipulation is pain relief (local anaesthesia).

Research suggests that acupuncture causes the release of heroin-like chemicals in the body which act as natural painkillers. Acupuncture can be effective in treating high blood pressure and can also overcome the effects of stress and encourage relaxation. Acupoints on the head, abdomen, trunk, back and foot are usually selected for stimulation, depending on your individual problem.

Acupressure is similar to acupuncture, but instead of inserting needles at selected points along the meridians, they are stimulated using firm thumb pressure or fingertip massage. The best-known example of acupressure is Shiatsu massage. This is particularly effective if combined with aromatherapy essential oils for a therapeutic massage. Best results are obtained if treatment is repeated three or four times a week.

AROMATHERAPY

Aromatherapy essential oils have powerful effects on your moods – the part of the brain (olfactory bulbs) that detects smell messages from the nose is closely linked with your emotional centre in the part of the brain called the limbic system. Oils are also absorbed from the skin into the circulation and can have powerful effects on the body. This is particularly noticeable in those oils that have diuretic properties.

Unless otherwise stated, aromatherapy oils should always be used in a diluted form by adding to a carrier oil – some neat oils will irritate body tissues. Use to massage into the skin, add to bathwater or diffuse into the air to scent your room.

Avoid using aromatherapy oils that are known to be capable of putting blood pressure up. These include thyme, clove and cinnamon.

Basil: helps to relieve stress (do not use during pregnancy)
Bergamot: helps to relieve stress
Birch: has diuretic properties; helps combat hardening and furring up of the arteries (atherosclerosis) (not during pregnancy)
Black Pepper: helps combat atherosclerosis
Cardamom: helps to relieve stress
Cedarwood: helps to relieve stress; has diuretic properties (not during pregnancy)
Chamomile: relaxing; helps to relieve stress; eases tension headaches; has diuretic properties (do not use during first 3 months of pregnancy)
Clary-sage: helps to lower high blood pressure; relaxing; helps to relieve stress (not during pregnancy)
Coriander: helps to relieve stress
Cypress: helps to relieve stress (not during pregnancy)
Eucalyptus: has diuretic properties
Fennel: helps to relieve stress; has diuretic properties
Geranium: helps to lower high blood pressure; relieves stress; eases tension headaches; has diuretic properties; helps coronary heart disease (CHD) (not during pregnancy)
Ginger: helps combat atherosclerosis

Grapefruit: helps to relieve stress
Jasmine: relaxing; helps to relieve stress (not during pregnancy)
Juniper: has diuretic properties; helps combat atherosclerosis
Lavender: helps to lower high blood pressure; relieves stress; eases tension headaches (not during first 3 months of pregnancy)
Lemon: helps to lower high blood pressure; has diuretic properties; helps combat atherosclerosis
Marjoram: helps to lower high blood pressure; relaxing; relieves stress (not during pregnancy)
Melissa: helps to lower high blood pressure
Neroli: helps to relieve stress
Nutmeg: helps to lower high blood pressure; relaxing (not during pregnancy)
Peppermint: eases tension headaches; has diuretic properties; helps CHD (not during pregnancy)
Pettigraine: relaxing
Rose: relaxing; helps to relieve stress (not during first 3 months of pregnancy)
Rosemary: helps to lower high blood pressure; eases tension headaches; helps combat atherosclerosis; helps CHD (not during pregnancy or if you suffer from epilepsy)
Rosewood: helps to relieve stress
Sandalwood: helps to relieve stress; has diuretic properties
Vetiver: relaxing; helps to relieve stress
Ylang ylang: helps to lower high blood pressure

If you suffer from fluid retention, don't use a diuretic oil for more than a day or two without seeking medical advice.

FLOATATION THERAPY

Floatation is a popular alternative therapy that can trigger profound relaxation. Paradoxically, it evolved from original studies in the 1950s designed to induce stress in humans. Few people could endure more than eight hours of water immersion and isolation (Restricted Environment Stimulation Therapy – also known as REST) and it was not until researchers experimented with floatation on salt solutions rather than complete water immersion, that the beneficial effects of floatation therapy were discovered.

Floatation therapy takes place in a light-proof, sound-insulated tank. This contains a shallow, 25-cm (10-inch) deep pool of warm saline in which 318 kg (700 lb) of Epsom Salts (magnesium sulphate) are dissolved to form a super-saturated solution more buoyant than the Dead Sea. The floater is suspended on this bed of minerals, which are kept at a constant skin temperature of 34.5°C (94.1°F). The tank is specially designed to screen out light and sound so the brain is cut off from virtually all external sources of stimulation – even the effects of gravity are minimized. This is probably important, as it has been suggested that 90 per cent of all brain activity is concerned with the effects of gravitational pull on the body (such as correcting posture, maintaining balance, etc.).

When brainwaves are recorded during relaxation, two patterns are seen: alpha and delta waves. Another pattern, theta waves, are more elusive and usually occur during deep meditation. Theta waves are accompanied by vivid memories, creative thought and feelings of serenity but are difficult to maintain without falling asleep. Studies at the University of Colorado have shown that during floatation therapy, your brain quickly starts generating theta waves while you remain awake – and what's more, you continue to make large amounts of creativity-promoting theta waves for up to three weeks after the float.

Many physiological changes occur throughout your body during floatation, including a significant fall in blood pressure in both normal and hypertensive people. A number of mechanisms are probably at work in producing this fall:

- blood levels of stress-inducing hormones (adrenaline, noradrenaline, cortisol and adrenocorticotrophic hormone) are reduced during repeated float sessions – this reduction is maintained even five days after treatment has stopped
- the parasympathetic nervous system is activated, which reduces heart rate, blood pressure, respiratory rate and sweating as well as relaxing muscles (including those in the

arteries and arteriolar walls) and oxygen requirements –
these effects are opposite to those of the fight-or-flight
(adrenaline) response linked with the sympathetic nervous
system

- secretion of anti-diuretic hormone decreases so that you
  produce larger quantities of urine shortly after a float,
  contributing to the fall in BP
- because sensory deprivation in a float tank allows the brain
  to focus in on the body (homeostatic feedback), most people
  can learn to slow their heart beat and blood pressure at will
  with a little practice
- increased levels of natural, heroin-like chemicals
  (endorphins and encephalins) are secreted in the brain
  during a float – these help relaxation and probably also
  explain the euphoria that many floaters feel.

In people with hypertension, even a single float lasting 45 minutes will lower BP. This effect continues gradually across repeated sessions, and the lower blood pressure is maintained after
floatation therapy stops. Control studies using subjects reclining
in dimly lit, quiet rooms do not show the same effects, so it is
not merely the process of relaxation that induces the measured
changes. As well as helping hypertension, floatation therapy
lowers raised cholesterol levels, relieves chronic pain and
reduces other unwanted effects of stress. Floating can also be
combined with audio tapes to enhance learning, for example of
a foreign language.

BIOFEEDBACK

Biofeedback is a technique – usually practised during meditation or during floatation therapy – in which adepts learn to
direct a body function that is not usually under voluntary control, such as speeding up or slowing the heart rate at will.
Research in the US suggests that 8 out of 10 people with hypertension can bring their blood pressure under control using a
simple biofeedback method. This involves placing a thermom-
eter on the floor and placing your bare foot on top of it so your

skin is in close contact with it. You then concentrate on your feet enough to raise your skin temperature to 36°C (96.8°F) – use mental images of your foot resting on a hot water bottle, and imagine your feet getting warmer and warmer. Biofeedback probably lowers BP by encouraging dilation of the peripheral circulation, including that in the skin – this opens up the circulation enough to let blood pressure fall.

HERBALISM

Phytotherapy – the use of plant extracts for healing – is one of the most exciting areas of medical research. Traditional herbs have provided orthodox medicine with many powerful drugs including aspirin (from the willow tree), digoxin (from the fox-glove) and even potent new cancer treatments such as paclitaxel (from the Pacific Yew tree). World-wide, specialists known as ethnobiologists are continually seeking new products from among the traditional herbs used by native healers. The Amazon has proved to be one of the richest sources, providing a wide range of traditional remedies.

Different parts of different plants are used – roots, stems, flowers, leaves, bark, sap, fruit or seeds – depending on which has the highest concentration of active ingredient. In most cases, these materials are dried and ground to produce a powder which is made into a tea, or packed into capsules for easy swallowing.

The following herbs all have medicinal uses to help high blood pressure. It is best to use them only after consulting a trained herbalist, and if you are having your blood pressure checked regularly by a medical doctor. Always check with both the herbalist and your usual doctor that any medications you are taking will not interact with any herbal prescriptions. Always inform your herbalist and your doctor of any other drugs you are taking – including ones bought over the counter – and take all medications exactly as prescribed. Never exceed the stated dose. Doses of each herb will vary depending on whether you are using dried preparations, tinctures, or extracts in the form of tablets or capsules. Always follow the dosage instructions on packets.

The plants used to treat heart problems often contain powerful chemicals called cardiac glycosides. These:

- stimulate contraction of heart muscle (the myocardium)
- improve the efficiency of the heart without increasing its oxygen needs
- increase cardiac output.

The most famous plant to contain cardiac glycosides is the foxglove (*digitalis*). Its active ingredients (such as digitoxin) have now been artificially synthesized and are used in orthodox medicines to treat a variety of heart problems. As its name implies, however, digitoxin is toxic at levels just above those needed for a therapeutic response, as they build up in the body and are not easily excreted. Natural foxglove is therefore not used by herbal practitioners.

The cardiac glycosides found in other herbs (such as Lily of the Valley) tend to be more easily excreted in the body and are less likely to produce toxic effects. However, you should not use these preparations without consulting a qualified herbalist first.

NB: Although Broom (*Cytisus scoparius*) is a herb commonly used to help the heart and for its diuretic action, you should not take it if you suffer from hypertension as it constricts peripheral vessels, which puts blood pressure up.

Buckwheat (*Fagopyrum esculentum*)

Buckwheat leaves are traditionally used to improve the tone of arteriolar walls and to help repair damage that may lead to atherosclerosis. It is sometimes used in the treatment of high blood pressure, especially that linked with retinal haemorrhage.

Black Haw (*Viburnum prunifolium*)

Dried bark from Black Haw, a close relative of Cramp Bark, helps to relax muscle tension and also has sedative actions, both of which explain its ability to lower blood pressure. Black Haw is also used:

- to help painful periods
- to treat threatened miscarriage or premature labour
- to help reduce bronchial spasm occurring in asthma.

Bugleweed (*Lycopus europaeus*)

The aerial parts (stems, leaves, sometimes the flowers) from Bugleweed increase the power of contraction of heart muscle, reduce the pulse rate and have a diuretic action. Bugleweed is used mainly to treat heart failure, especially where this is due to high blood pressure or an overactive thyroid gland. It is also used as a sedative and anti-cough remedy.

Cramp Bark (*Viburnum opulus*)

Cramp Bark (the guelder rose), as its name suggests, is used to reduce muscle tension and spasm. This relaxant action also occurs in the smooth muscles lining the peripheral blood vessels. It also has a sedative action which can reduce the effects of stress. Both actions help to reduce high blood pressure. Cramp Bark is also used:

- to help painful periods
- to reduce blood loss linked with heavy periods, especially around the menopause
- to treat threatened miscarriage.

Chrysanthemum (*Chrysanthemum morifolium*)

Chrysanthemum flowers (Ju Hua) are used in Chinese medicine to dilate the coronary arteries, improve blood flow through heart muscle and boost cardiac output. As heart function improves, treatment can reduce and stabilize high blood pressure. Chrysanthemum flowers are also used for their cooling and anti-microbial actions.

Dandelion (*Taraxacum officinalis*)

Dandelion is a powerful diuretic as well as being a rich source of the mineral potassium. It helps to flush excess sodium salts and fluid through the kidneys and is so effective that in mediaeval times it was known as 'piss-a-bed'. It is a useful treatment for high blood pressure as it can reduce fluid retention without also encouraging a build-up of sodium. Interestingly, dandelion does not seem to have a diuretic action in those with a normal healthy fluid balance who do not need to lose excess water. Dandelion is also used:

- to stimulate bile flow
- to boost the metabolic rate
- to aid digestion
- as a laxative
- as a tonic
- to relieve rheumatic pains.

Figwort (*Scrophularia nodosa*)

The aerial parts of Figwort are known mainly for their beneficial effects against a variety of skin complaints including eczema, psoriasis and itching. It also acts as a mild laxative and as an anti-inflammatory antibiotic (originally used to treat scrofula – tuberculosis involving lymph glands in the neck, hence its Latin name). The root of the Chinese Figwort, *S. ningpoensis*, is used to increase the strength of heart muscle contraction, to lower high blood pressure and for its mild diuretic action.

NB: Figwort should not be used if the heart beat is abnormally fast (above 100 beats per minute).

Garlic (*Allium sativum*)

Garlic has a number of medicinal uses, of which the most important are its ability to reduce the risk of CHD and stroke. Research shows that taking tablets containing standardized extracts of dried, powdered garlic (600–900 mg per day) can:

- lower high blood pressure enough to reduce the risk of a stroke by up to 40 per cent
- reduce harmful blood fat levels (LDL-cholesterol and triglycerides) by 12 per cent
- reduce the risk of blood clots
- decrease blood stickiness and improve circulation to parts of the body by 48 per cent
- reduce blood glucose (sugar) levels
- reduce the risk of a dangerous heart rhythm
- reduce the risk of CHD by up to 25 per cent
- improve blood flow to the brain, improving memory and concentration.

Garlic also has antiseptic, antibacterial and antiviral properties and is commonly used to treat respiratory infections and skin warts. Garlic products made by solvent extraction or by boiling in oil are less effective than tablets made from garlic that has been freeze-dried and powdered, which retains more of the active ingredients (*see Chapter 10*).

Ginkgo (*Ginkgo biloba*)

Ginkgo leaves contain unique chemicals – ginkgosides – that improve blood flow throughout the body, especially the brain, hands and feet. Ginkgo supplements can help to improve peripheral circulation that has been hampered due to hardening and furring up of the arteries. It is particularly useful for those with pain in one or both calves brought on by exercise (intermittent claudication due to lack of blood and oxygen reaching the calf muscles). Ginkgo is also used to treat:

- irregular heart beat
- leg ulcers
- varicose veins
- haemorrhoids
- chilblains
- poor memory and concentration
- dizziness

- tinnitus
- anxiety.

Hawthorn (*Crategus oxycantha* and *C. monogyna*)

The flowering tops and berries of the Hawthorn are among the most beneficial herbal remedies available for treating the heart and circulation. They contain chemicals that normalize the cardiovascular system, either relaxing or stimulating it as necessary, and may therefore be used in the treatment of opposing problems. Hawthorn helps to reduce high blood pressure by:

- relaxing peripheral blood vessels
- dilating the coronary arteries, improving blood circulation to heart muscle
- discouraging fluid retention
- slowing and possibly even reversing the build-up of atheromatous plaques.

It also increases the strength and efficiency of the heart's pumping action. Hawthorn preparations are so effective in helping angina and hypertension that more research on Hawthorn is currently underway.

Horsetail (*Equisetum arvense*)

The dried stems from Horsetail have a mild diuretic action and also improve muscular tone throughout the urinary tract. Horsetail is used to reduce fluid retention and treat a number of urinary problems such as recurrent cystitis, benign prostate disease, stress incontinence and childhood bedwetting. It is also used to:

- staunch bleeding and hasten wound healing
- reduce blood loss in heavy periods
- improve the circulation
- treat skin conditions.

Huang Qi (*Astragalus membranaceus*)

Astragalus root (Huang Qi) is used in Chinese medicine as a cardiotonic and diuretic, sometimes recommended in the treatment of high blood pressure.

Lemon Balm (*Melissa officinalis*)

Lemon balm is a healing herb with calming properties. Its leaves are widely used to combat the effects of nervous stress, to improve heart function and for their blood pressure-lowering effects. It is also used to help relieve:

- spasm of the intestinal tract
- nausea and flatulence
- depression
- headache
- feverish conditions (such as influenza)
- insomnia.

Lily of the Valley (*Convallaria majalis*)

Dried Lily of the Valley leaves contain a number of powerful cardiac glycosides, two of which act directly on the heart. They have a similar action to digitoxin (from the Foxglove) but without the potentially dangerous side-effects. Lily of the Valley is used to help treat:

- angina
- hardening and furring up of the arteries (atherosclerosis)
- water retention due to heart failure
- heart failure associated with high blood pressure.

Lime Blossom (*Tilia vulgaris*)

Dried flowers from the Lime Blossom (or Linden) tree have an anti-atheroma action similar to that of garlic. If used long term, this herb can help to prevent furring up of the arteries and may even reduce the amount of atheroma already present. It is widely used to lower high blood pressure and to reduce the effects of nervous tension. Its anti-hypertensive effect seems to be due to relaxation and dilation of blood vessels, which also makes it helpful in the relief of some forms of migraine. It also promotes sweating, making it useful for treating feverish conditions such as influenza.

Mistletoe (*Viscum alba*)

Mistletoe leaves and twigs (not the berries, which are poisonous) has a direct action on the vagus nerve (a cranial nerve stretching from the brain down to the heart and chest) to slow the heart rate. It also strengthens the walls of small blood vessels (capillaries) and has anti-atherosclerosis action. It can lower blood pressure significantly, and is also used to ease headache associated with high BP.

Motherwort (*Leonurus cardiaca*)

The leaves of Motherwort have been used since Roman times to strengthen heart muscle, ease palpitations, regulate a fast pulse and lower raised blood pressure.

Motherwort is also used to:

- ease anxiety and nervous tension
- stimulate menstrual flow
- relieve period pains
- bring on a period delayed by emotional shock
- relieve menopausal hot flushes.

As it is a uterine stimulant, it is not usually advised during pregnancy (with the exception of labour).

Night-blooming Cereus (*Selenicereus grandiflorus*)

Fresh stems from the Night-blooming Cereus have a similar action on the heart to Lily of the Valley. This herb is used to treat mild heart failure, water retention, shortness of breath and palpitations. It does not contain cardiac glycosides.

Paeony (*Paeonia* spp)

Paeony root is used to stimulate the circulation, reduce high blood pressure, relieve pain and as a sedative. It also has antibacterial and anti-inflammatory actions and has proved useful in the treatment of eczema.

Skullcap (*Scutellaria laterifolia*)

Leaves and flowers from the skullcap are widely used to treat stress and related problems including nervous tension, hysteria, exhaustion and depression. It can also be used to help treat epilepsy and pre-menstrual syndrome. It can help to lower high blood pressure linked with acute stress.

Squill (*Urginea maritima*)

Squill contains cardiac glycosides which stimulate the heart, and is used to help treat congestive heart failure and associated water retention (that is, secondary to high blood pressure). Only a minute quantity of the bulb is prescribed; this is usually given in the form of a dilute tincture. It also acts to thin mucus secretions and is used as an expectorant to relieve dry cough or excess sticky mucus (such as in chronic bronchitis).

Valerian (*Valeriana officinalis*)

Valerian roots contain a natural sedative that make it one of the most relaxing herbs available. It has significant, positive effects on stress and as well as relieving anxiety and tension; it induces sleep, eases smooth muscle spasm and promotes calmness. It is used to lower high blood pressure, especially where this is linked with stress. Valerian can also relieve cramps, period pains, intestinal colic, migraine, rheumatic pains and some types of epilepsy.

Wood Betony (*Stachys officinalis*)

The aerial parts of Wood Betony have a sedative action and are used to treat nervous tension. It is a relaxant and painkiller useful for treating the tension headache linked with stress and raised blood pressure.

Yarrow (*Achillea millefolium*)

Aerial parts from Yarrow contain chemicals that lower a raised blood pressure by encouraging dilation of peripheral blood vessels and through its diuretic action. It also has an anti-atheroma action and is commonly recommended to help treat thrombotic conditions linked with high blood pressure. Yarrow is also used:

- to help cystitis
- to encourage wound healing
- to stimulate digestion
- to promote sweating and lower a fever.

HOMOEOPATHY

Homoeopathic medicine is based on the belief that natural substances can boost the body's own healing powers to relieve the symptoms and signs of illness. Natural substances are selected which, if used full-strength, would produce symptoms in a healthy person similar to those it is designed to treat. This is the first principle of homoeopathy, that 'Like cures Like.'

The second major principle of homoeopathy is that increasing the dilution of a solution has the opposite effect, that is, increases its potency ('Less Cures More'). By diluting noxious and even poisonous substances many millions of times, their healing properties are enhanced while their undesirable side-effects are lost.

On the centesimal scale, dilutions of 100^{-6} (1 drop tincture mixed with 99 drops alcohol or water and shaken; this is then done a further six times, each time 1 drop of the dilution being added to 99 drops of alcohol or water) are described as potencies of 6C, dilutions of 100^{-30} are written as a potency of 30C, etc. To illustrate just how diluted these substances are, a dilution of 12C (100^{-12}) is comparable to a pinch of salt dissolved in the same amount of water as is found in the Atlantic Ocean!

Homoeopathy is thought to work in a dynamic way, boosting your body's own healing powers. The principles that like cures like and less cures more are difficult concepts to accept, yet convincing trials have shown that homoeopathy is significantly better than placebos in treating many chronic (long-term) conditions including hayfever, asthma and rheumatoid arthritis.

Homoeopathic remedies should ideally be taken on their own, at least 30 minutes either before or after eating or drinking. Tablets should also be taken without handling them first – tip them into the lid of the container, or onto a teaspoon to transfer them into your mouth. Then suck or chew them, don't swallow them whole.

Homoeopathic treatments are prescribed according to your symptoms rather than any particular disease, so two people with the same health problem will usually need different homoeopathic treatments.

Homoeopathic remedies may be prescribed by a medically-trained homoeopathic doctor on a normal NHS prescription form and dispensed by homoeopathic pharmacists for the usual prescription charge or exemption. Alternatively, you can consult a private homoeopathic practitioner or buy remedies direct from the pharmacist.

Although it is best to see a trained homoeopath who can assess your constitutional type, personality, lifestyle, family background, likes and dislikes as well as your symptoms before deciding which treatment is right for you, you may find the following remedies helpful.

After taking the remedies for the time stated, if there is no obvious improvement consult a practitioner. Don't be surprised if your symptoms initially get worse before they get better – persevere through this common reaction to treatment – it is a good sign which shows the remedy is working.

There are no specific homoeopathic remedies to treat hypertension. Those used to help circulatory disorders and the effects of excess stress may prove beneficial, however.

■ For arteriolar spasm leading to poor peripheral blood flow, especially in the hands and feet on exposure to cold; also for

headaches that are worse in the morning: *Carbo. veg 6C*.
(Take every 30 minutes for up to 10 doses)
- For tension headache that comes on suddenly and feel like a
tight band round the head: *Aconite 30C*.
(Take every 10 minutes for up to 10 doses)
- For tension headache brought on by emotional stress – a
sharp severe pain in the side of the head accompanied by
the 'tight band' sensation: *Ignatia 30C*.
(Take every 10 minutes for up to 10 doses)
- For a tension headache that feels bursting and crushing,
with sharp pain brought on by the slightest eye movement:
Byronia 30C. (Take every 10 minutes for up to 10 doses)
- For tension headache with muscular spasm and stiffness in
the neck: *Cimic. 6C*. (Take every hour for up to 5 doses)

MASSAGE

Massage is one of the oldest complementary therapies known to
humanity. Massage is particularly useful to help tension, circulatory problems, high blood pressure, insomnia, depression,
back pain and muscular aches. There are many different types
of massage which use a variety of rubbing, drumming, knead-
ing, friction and pressure strokes. All are very relaxing.

MEDITATION

Meditation is a self-help technique in which the power of concentration is used to control thoughts, and to calm the body.
Those experienced in meditation enter a trance-like state; some
can lower their pulse and blood pressure at will (*see Biofeedback
and Floatation Therapy, above*). Muscular tension drops, circulation improves and brain wave patterns change. Meditation
often leads to sleep.

For those who find meditation difficult, a so-called Mind
Machine may help. These relatively new devices can help you
alter your brainwave patterns within a few minutes to produce any mood you are looking for, including deeply relaxing

rhythms which are usually only achievable with many years' practice.

Your brainwaves naturally vary according to your mental state:

- beta rhythms (14 cycles/sec) occur when your mind is busy and buzzing
- alpha rhythms (8–13 cycles/sec) make you feel elated, calm and in a meditative state
- theta-waves (4–8 cycles/sec) cause deep relaxation and creative bursts of thought
- delta waves (below 4 cycles/sec) occur in deep, dreamless sleep (and during floatation therapy).

Using a Mind Machine lets you select one of these states with ease. You put on special goggles that produce flickering light rhythms, and headphones that produce repetitive sounds. The patterns start off by reproducing beta wave (wakeful) rhythms, then slowly change to trigger other states. Your mind responds to powerful, repetitive rhythms and will soon start to mimic them, changing its brainwave pattern to follow the rhythm it is exposed to. You can use the Mind Machine to produce relaxation, sleep, to energize you, to increase your learning power, and to tap into your creativity before writing, painting or composing music. For someone with high blood pressure, selecting a relaxing rhythm will quickly take you down through the alpha state and into a profoundly relaxed, theta state.

REFLEXOLOGY

Reflexology is based on the principle that points in the feet – known as reflexes – are directly related to other parts of the body. Massage over these reflexes can detect areas of tenderness and subtle textural changes which help to pinpoint problems in various organs. By working on these tender spots with tiny pressure movements, nerves are thought to be stimulated that pass messages to distant organs and relieve symptoms. Some people with hypertension have found reflexology helpful.

YOGA

This ancient Oriental technique involves postural exercises, breathing techniques and relaxation. It is excellent for improving joint suppleness, relieving stress and reducing high blood pressure.

Chapter Ten

LIFESTYLE AND DIETARY CHANGES

BP AND YOUR LIFESTYLE

One of the main causes of high blood pressure is hardening and narrowing of the arteries. This naturally occurs with increasing age and comes on more quickly if you smoke or are overweight. Other lifestyle factors that can raise your blood pressure include drinking too much alcohol, being under excessive stress, lack of exercise and possibly drinking too much caffeine – especially when you are under stress.

New evidence suggests that doctors may be able to predict which people with hypertension will respond best to losing weight and reducing their salt intake. This involves measuring blood levels of circulating renin. Renin hormone is made in the kidney and acts to put blood pressure up (*see page 15*). For people with high renin levels, weight loss is three times more effective in reducing blood pressure than in those with low renin levels – the former also respond better to a low-sodium, high-potassium diet.

SUGGESTED LIFESTYLE CHANGES FOR PEOPLE WITH HYPERTENSION

- If you smoke, try to stop – chemicals in cigarettes damage artery linings, cause spasm and constriction of vessels, and raise your blood pressure.
- Do not drink excessive amounts of alcohol, although moderate intakes seem to be protective.
- Try to avoid stressful situations and take time out to relax – stress hormones send BP rocketing. Try floatation therapy, or have an

aromatherapy bath with oils of Lavender, Marjoram or Ylang Ylang (*see Chapter 9*).
- Watch your caffeine intake, especially if you are under stress.
- Women should consider taking HRT after the menopause.
- Lose any excess weight – this can sometimes lower blood pressure enough to bring it back down to normal and get you off treatment.
- Increase the amount of exercise you take – try to walk as much as possible, and use the stairs instead of the lift.
- Eat a healthy diet with plenty of fresh fruit and vegetables for protective vitamins, minerals and fibre.
- Cut back on your salt intake by not adding it during cooking or at the table.
- If you have diabetes, make sure your blood sugar levels are well controlled.

HOW DIET AND LIFESTYLE CHANGES REDUCE YOUR RISK OF CORONARY HEART DISEASE (CHD)

Factor modified	Reduction in risk of CHD
Stopping smoking:	50–70 per cent lower risk within 5 years
Keeping alcohol intakes within healthy limits:	25–45 per cent lower risk for those drinking 2–3 units per day
Taking HRT:	44 per cent lower risk after the menopause
Losing excess weight:	35–55 per cent lower risk for those who maintain a healthy weight
Exercise:	45 per cent lower risk for those who exercise regularly
Reducing blood cholesterol levels:	2–3 per cent lower risk for each 1 per cent reduction through exercise, diet or medication
Taking prophylactic aspirin:	33 per cent lower risk in users compared with non-users (*see Chapter 8*)
Controlling high blood pressure:	2–3 per cent lower risk for each 1 mmHg reduction of diastolic BP

Smoking

Smoking cigarettes is linked with early death from a number of illnesses, including CHD, high blood pressure and stroke. If you can give up, your health will quickly benefit:

- within 20 minutes: your blood pressure and pulse rate will fall significantly as arterial spasm decreases
- within 8 hours: levels of carbon monoxide in your blood drop to normal so that blood oxygen levels can rise
- within 48 hours: the stickiness of your blood and the quantity of blood-clotting factors present will fall enough to reduce your risk of a heart attack or stroke
- within 1–3 months: the blood supply to your peripheries will increase, and your lung function will improve by up to a third
- within 5 years: your risk of lung cancer will have halved
- within 10 years: your risk of all smoking-related cancers (such as of the lung, mouth, throat, bladder) will have reduced to almost normal levels.

Tips on How to Stop Smoking

- Get into the right frame of mind.
- Name the day to give up.
- Try to stop at the same time as a friend or relative for support.
- Throw away all smoking bits and pieces such as matches, lighters, ashtrays, etc.
- Take it one day at a time and just concentrate on getting through each day.
- Keep a chart and tick off each successful day.
- Find something to occupy your hands, such as making models, drawing or origami.
- Take extra exercise.
- When you have an urge to smoke, try sucking on celery or carrot sticks, eating an apple, or cleaning your teeth with strong flavoured toothpaste.
- Avoid situations where you used to smoke.
- Learn to say 'No thanks, I've given up.'
- Ask friends and relatives not to smoke around you.

Alcohol

A moderate intake of alcohol – especially red wine – can lower your blood pressure, reduce stress levels and decrease your risk of CHD by 25–45 per cent. This is mostly due to the powerful antioxidants found in red wine, and the thinning effect of alcohol on the blood. New research shows that if you have hypertension and drink within the recommended limits, your risk of dying from a stroke is 40 per cent less than someone with hypertension who is tee-total.

If you drink excessive amounts of alcohol, however, it can significantly increase your blood pressure, increase your risk of CHD and stroke as well as damaging your liver, leading to cirrhosis. Men who drink more than 6 units of alcohol in one session are at twice the risk of sudden death than those who drink moderately (2–4 units):

■ men should aim to drink no more than 3–4 units of alcohol per day, with an average weekly intake of 21 units considered the safe maximum
■ women should drink no more than 2–3 units per day, with an average weekly limit of 14 units.

1 unit of alcohol is equivalent to:

■ 100 ml (1 glass) of wine, or
■ 50 ml (one measure) of sherry, or
■ 25 ml (one tot) of spirit, or
■ 300 ml (half a pint) of normal strength beer.

For men, drinking more than 50 units of alcohol per week is considered dangerous, while for women, the equivalent figure is 35 units. If you have hypertension and regularly drink above the maximum recommended safe limit, it is important that you cut back. Simple tips to help you cut back on your alcohol intake include:

■ When drinking alcohol, sip slowly and keep putting your glass down rather than holding it in your hand – this will reduce the amount you drink.
■ Savour each sip and hold it in your mouth for longer than you normally would.
■ Alternate each alcoholic drink with a non-alcoholic one.

- Many bars offer exotic, non-alcoholic cocktails such as mango juice with coconut milk which are delicious and full of nutrients.
- Drink mineral water with a dash of fresh lemon juice, or low-calorie drinks.
- Tonic water with ice, lemon and a dash of Angostura bitters is an excellent substitute for a gin and tonic.
- Mix chilled white or red wine with sparkling mineral water to make a refreshing spritzer.
- Drink fruit/herbal teas – these are delicious, relaxing or stimulating depending on which you choose and, as they are drunk without milk, have the additional bonus of being calorie-free.
- Elderflower cordial diluted with mineral water is an excellent substitute for white wine.

Stress

Stress is the term used to describe being under too much pressure. A certain amount of stress is good for you and helps you to meet life's challenges, but too much is harmful. When you are stressed, your pulse and blood pressure go up significantly. In a recent study looking at almost 300 male employees in the US, those reporting high levels of work stress had much greater BPs – the effect was equivalent to carrying an extra 18 kg (40 lb) in weight, or an additional 20 years in age.

Stress is harmful because it can trigger:

- high blood pressure and stroke
- arterial spasm, chest pain, angina and heart attack
- palpitations, a racing pulse and an irregular heart rhythm
- over-breathing (hyperventilation)
- dizziness, faintness and trembling
- sensations of pins and needles, numbness
- headache
- sweating and flushing
- tiredness and fatigue
- stomach pains and peptic ulcers
- nausea and nervous diarrhoea

- insomnia and bad dreams
- increased susceptibility to infections
- emotional problems such as anxiety and depression.

If you suffer from hypertension, it is important to reduce your stress levels. In some people, stress can trigger overactivity of the sympathetic nervous system, causing large daily swings in your BP. This is known as labile hypertension or Gaisbock's syndrome, and increases your risk of developing future sustained hypertension (*see Chapter 3*) and of suffering a stroke.

If you suffer from high blood pressure, feel stressed, or develop any of the stress-related symptoms listed above, it is important to see your doctor.

Tips to Help Overcome Stress

- Try to slow down and relax.
- Work out what is making you stressed and why – change those situations that can be changed and, where practical, avoid others (such as shopping in the supermarket at the busiest times).
- Leave more time for tasks so they aren't done under deadline pressure.
- Learn to say 'no' so you are not put upon by others.
- Exercise regularly to burn off stress hormones.
- Try floatation therapy (*see page 85*).
- Increase your intake of vitamins C and the B group, as these are rapidly used up by stress reactions in your body.
  - Vitamin C is found in fresh fruit and vegetables, especially citrus fruits.
  - Vitamin B is found in wholegrain cereals, dark green vegetables and yeast extract, as well as meat and dairy products.
- Cut back on sugar, salt and excess fat.
- Eat little and often to keep your blood sugar constant.
- If you smoke, try to cut back or stop.
- Keep alcohol intake within the low-risk range.
- Avoid drinks and products containing caffeine.

Caffeine

Caffeine is a drug that can put your BP up and worsen the effects of high stress levels or a high-salt diet. In one study, assessing the effect of coffee on blood pressure in over 10,000 American males during a 32-year period, a positive link was found between coffee intake and hypertension. The risk of developing high blood pressure was three times greater in those drinking five or more cups of coffee daily compared to those who did not drink coffee.

Taking HRT after the Female Menopause

Before the menopause, women enjoy some protection against atherosclerosis, high blood pressure and CHD, as the female hormone oestrogen acts on artery walls to keep them healthy and elastic. After the menopause, however, falling oestrogen levels encourage hardening and furring up of the arteries plus high blood pressure, so that a woman's risk of CHD rapidly rises. By taking hormone replacement therapy (HRT), the beneficial effects of oestrogen can be enjoyed for longer. Studies show that taking HRT can reduce the risk of CHD in post-menopausal women by up to 50 per cent. If a woman has already had a heart attack, HRT provides 80 per cent protection against another occurring. In women for whom it is suitable, the benefits of taking HRT for up to 10 years (from the age of 50) more than outweigh the risks – that is, it provides maximum protection against CHD and osteoporosis, with a minimum risk of causing breast cancer. Ask your doctor for further advice.

Losing Weight

Being overweight significantly increases your risk of many diseases, including high blood pressure, CHD, and stroke. Excess fat (adipose tissue) increases the resistance against which your heart has to pump blood out into your general circulation. People who are overweight are also more likely to be eating excess fat, to have high blood cholesterol and glucose levels, and to take little in the way of regular exercise. All these factors hasten atherosclerosis and are likely to put your blood pressure up.

Are You in the Healthy Weight Range for Your Height?

The best way to work out if you are in the healthy weight range for your height is to determine your body mass index (BMI). This is calculated by dividing your weight (in kilograms) by the square of your height (in metres).

BMI = Weight (kg) ÷ Height × Height (M²)

The calculation produces a number that can be interpreted by the following table:

BMI WEIGHT BAND

Less than 20	Underweight
20–25	Healthy
25–30	Overweight
30–40	Obese
More than 40	Morbidly Obese

A BMI of 20–25 is in the healthy weight range, as it is not linked with an increased risk of early death. The following chart does the calculating for you:

HEALTHY WEIGHT RANGES FOR HEIGHT

Height (metres/ft)	Optimum Healthy Weight Range (kg/stones):	
	Men	Women
1.52/5 ft		43–55/6 st 11 8 st 9
1.55/5'1"		45–57/7 st 1–8 st 13
1.57/5'2"		46–59/7 st 3–9 st 4
1.60/5'3"		48–61/7 st 8–9 st 8
1.63/5'4"		50–63/7 st 12–9 st 13
1.65/5'5"		51–65/8 st–10 st 3
1.68/5'6"	56–70/8 st 12–11 st	53–67/8 st 5–10 st 7
1.70/5'7"	58–72/9 st 1–11 st 4	54–69/8 st 7–10 st 12
1.73/5'8"	60–75/9 st 6–11 st 10	56–71/8 st 11–11 st 2
1.75/5'9"	61–76/9 st 9–12 st	57–73/8 st 13–11 st 7
1.78/5'10"	63–79/9 st 13–12 st 6	59–75/9 st 4–11 st 1
1.80/5'11"	65–81/10 st 3–12 st 9	61–77/9 st 8–12 st 1
1.83/6 ft	67–83/10 st 7–13 st 1	63–80/9 st 13–12 st 8
1.85/6'1"	69–85/10 st 11–13 st 5	
1.88/6'2"	71–88/11 st 2–13 st 12	
1.90/6'3"	72–90/11 st 5–14 st 2	
1.93/6'4"	75–93/11 st 10–14 st 8	

If your BMI falls above this range, you are either overweight (BMI of 25–30) or obese (BMI of 30–40 or more). Overweight increases your risk of premature death from high blood pressure, CHD or stroke by 50 per cent. If you are obese, your risk of premature death from these causes is double that of someone who is in the healthy weight range for his or her height.

Where you store your excess fat is also important. Overweight people who carry excess weight around their middle (apple-shaped) rather than around their hips (pear-shaped) are at greater risk of CHD, stroke, high blood pressure, atherosclerosis, raised cholesterol levels and diabetes.

If you are overweight and are also apple-shaped, you have a significantly high risk of developing high blood pressure and CHD and should seriously consider losing at least some of your excess weight. Shedding just 3.2 kg (half a stone) can produce a significant fall in high blood pressure.

How to Lose Weight

The only way to lose weight is to eat fewer calories than you burn. The most successful way to do this is to lose only around 0.5–1 kg (1–2 lb) per week. If you try to lose weight more quickly, your health may suffer. You are also less likely to lose weight and keep it off – your metabolism is designed to conserve energy in the face of possible impending starvation and will slow right down, so you shed excess fat more slowly and painfully. Once you start eating normally again, your metabolism will stay on its super-efficient setting and the weight will pile back on.

Most experts now agree that you need to:

■ follow a low-fat diet to take off excess weight
■ exercise regularly to keep the weight off.

Healthy Eating and Weight Loss Plan for Someone with Hypertension

The following healthy eating plan can be followed whether or not you have excess weight to lose. It guides your food choices and encourages you to eat more unrefined complex carbohydrates, fruit, vegetables and fibre. It also lowers your fat intake and can help you to reduce your risk of hypertension and CHD while maintaining a healthy weight, or losing excess fat. Most people who have followed the weight-loss part of this diet have dropped the pounds easily without suffering from hunger pangs. If you do feel peckish, eat an extra slice of brown bread/toast, an extra piece of fruit or a low-fat yoghurt.

Every day you are allowed to eat a set number of units from five different food groups:

1. complex carbohydrates
2. fruits and vegetables
3. dairy products
4. fish, pulses, nuts and seeds
5. meat and eggs.

Within each food group, a range of intakes is allowed depending on whether you want to maintain your current weight while eating more healthily, or to lose excess weight.

Within each plan a range of intakes is given for each food type. If you are relatively inactive, stick to the bottom end of the unit range when selecting how much food you can eat. Then, on days when you are more active and/or taking part in an exercise programme, you can eat more and select your unit intake from the upper end of the range, especially within the complex carbohydrate group.

When selecting your daily unit allowance, make sure you obtain a wide variety of foods. Some are higher in calories than others but, over a period of time, your calorie intake will average out.

How to Follow the Diet

1. Turn to Chart 1 (*page 13*) to find out how many units you can eat from each food group per day, depending on whether you are male or female, and whether you want to maintain your weight while eating more healthily, or to lose excess weight.
2. Add in your daily allowances (Chart 2, *page 13*).
3. Look at the food unit groups (Chart 3, *page 14*) to see which foods you can choose from in each group.
4. Write your daily unit allowance at the top of your daily unit record (Chart 4, *page 13*), then write in the number of units you have eaten after each meal or snack. This will help you keep track of the units you've had, and how many you still have left.

CHART 1: DAILY UNITS ALLOWED FROM EACH FOOD GROUP

Men

Units of Each Food Group Allowed Per Day

	Carbohydrate	Veg	Dairy	Fish	Meat
Healthy Eating Plan	8–10	6–12	2–3	2–4	0–1
Weight Loss Plan	4–7	5–10	1–2	1–2	0–1

Women

Units of Each Food Group Allowed Per Day

	Carbohydrate	Veg	Dairy	Fish	Meat
Healthy Eating Plan	5–7	5–10	2–3	2–3	0–1
Weight Loss Plan	3–5	5–8	1–2	1–2	0–1

CHART 2: DAILY ALLOWANCES

As well as the number of units you can choose from each of the food groups, you can add in several additional allowances each day. These are:

- 300 ml ($^1/_2$ pint) skimmed or semi-skimmed milk
- Tea or coffee using your milk allowance or additional milk units. Limit yourself to a total of 3 cups per day and try not to use sugar or sweeteners.
- 15 g ($^1/_2$ oz) butter or spread made from olive oil or rapeseed oil per day
- a scraping of low-sugar, high-fruit diet jam/marmalade or yeast extract
- light brushing with olive oil while grilling or baking fish or meat
- as many fresh herbs and spices as you wish
- as much fresh lemon or lime juice as you wish
- as many milk-free herbal/fruit teas as you wish
- as much mineral water as you wish – sparkling, plain or with an added twist of fresh lemon or lime juice. Try to drink 3 litres ($4^1/_2$ pints) of fluid per day.
- try not to add salt to food while cooking or at the table – use black pepper and fresh herbs/spices for flavouring instead
- 1 glass (100 ml) of wine (preferably red) or red grape juice

with your evening meal – but try not to drink more than this while following the weight loss plan

■ a multinutrient supplement containing vitamins and minerals; garlic powder tablets (Kwai is recommended); omega-3 fish oil supplements.

CHART 3: WHAT THE FOOD UNITS IN EACH GROUP CONSIST OF

1 unit equals any of the following items:

1. Complex carbohydrates

6 tablespoons any unsweetened breakfast cereal
2 medium slices wholemeal or brown bread/toast
1 wholemeal bread roll
1 wholemeal pitta bread
1 medium chapatti
1 slice fruity malt loaf
1 slice rye bread
1 slice pumpernickel bread
$^1/_4$ French stick bread
4 slimmer's crispbreads
2 plain/digestive biscuits
4 tablespoons (100 g) cooked brown rice
1 cupful (100 g) cooked pasta (such as wholemeal or flavoured with spinach; herbs and garlic; sun-dried tomatoes, etc.)
2 medium boiled potatoes
1 large baked potato

2. Fruits and vegetables

small glass (100 ml) freshly squeezed fruit juice
serving of low-fat vegetable soup, etc.
sauce made with tomato juice, herbs, orange juice, etc.
1 generous serving (as much as you want) of any fresh green vegetable (such as spinach, broccoli, green beans, garden peas, etc.)
large mixed-leaf salad sprinkled with nuts and seeds

1 serving of fresh root vegetable such as carrot, parsnip
1 large beef tomato or 2 medium tomatoes
1 apple, orange, kiwi, peach, pear, nectarine, small banana
$^1/_2$ grapefruit, $^1/_2$ ogen melon, $^1/_2$ mango, $^1/_2$ papaya
2 dates, figs (fresh or dried), satsumas
4 passion fruit, apricots, plums, prunes
1 generous serving (100 g) fresh strawberries, raspberries, blackberries, redcurrants, etc.
a handful (100 g) of grapes, cherries
2 fresh pineapple rings (100 g)
1 serving (100 g) minimally sweetened rhubarb, gooseberries

3. Dairy products

200 ml ($^1/_3$ pint) semi-skimmed milk
300 ml ($^1/_2$ pint) skimmed milk
30 g (1 oz) hard cheese
60 g (2 oz) reduced fat cheese
small carton (150 g) of very low-fat cottage cheese
small carton (150 g) very low-fat natural fromage frais
small carton (150 g) natural BIO yoghurt
Ideally, add chopped, fresh fruit to natural yoghurt rather than eating sweetened, flavoured ones.

4. Fish, pulses, nuts and seeds

small fillet (50 g) oily fish
medium fillet (100 g) non-oily white fish
1 small tin of tuna in olive oil (drained)
1 serving (100 g) lobster or crab meat
1 serving (100 g) peeled prawns, scampi, shrimps
1 pint (400 g) fresh mussels (400 g)
1 serving (100 g) cooked lentils, haricot beans, baked beans, kidney beans, chick peas, etc.
8 walnut halves (or similar)
2–3 tablespoons mixed seeds

5. Meat and eggs

2 eggs (size 4), boiled or poached (maximum of 3–4 eggs per week)

1 egg = $1/2$ unit and still falls within the 0–1 unit allowance – you don't *have* to eat 2!

2 slices lean ham

1 small portion (75 g) minced meat

2 slices (75 g) lean red meat, all visible fat removed

2 slices well-cooked duck with skin removed

3 slices (100 g) chicken without skin

Record what you eat during the day, work out how many units it contains, and make sure you don't eat more than your allotted allowance. This is most easily done by photocopying the daily unit record (Chart 4, *page 17*) and filling it in after every meal.

Working Out the Units in a Meal

The anti-hypertensive diet is designed to help you eat more healthily with a minimum of fuss and bother. As long as you stick to the number of units you are allowed, you can continue to eat most of your favourite foods and even select foods from restaurants when eating out. It will adapt to fit almost any lifestyle.

It is easy to estimate how much of each food group you are eating. For example:

If you have a meal of carrot and orange soup, spaghetti with tuna and tomato sauce, salad and garlic bread followed by an apple, cheese and biscuits, the unit content works out as follows:

carrot and orange soup: 1–2 units veg (depending on size of portion)

pasta: 2 units complex carbohydrate (depends on how large a portion you have. Get to know roughly what 1 unit – 100 g – of cooked pasta looks like)

tuna and tomato sauce: 1 unit veg (onions and tomato in sauce); 1 unit fish

salad: 1 unit vegetables; small amount olive oil for dressing
from allowance
garlic bread: 1 unit carbohydrate ($^1/_4$ French stick); plus
butter from allowance
apple: 1 unit fruit
cheese (60 g): 2 units dairy
biscuits: 1 unit carbohydrate.

This meal has cost you the following number of units:

Complex Carbohydrates:	4
Vegetables and Fruit:	4–5
Dairy Products:	2
Fish, beans, seeds and nuts:	1
Meat and Eggs:	0

CHART 4: RECORD OF UNITS EATEN FROM EACH GROUP PER DAY

	Carbohydrates	Fruit/Veg	Dairy	Fish/Pulses	Meat/Eggs
Total Allowed per day	[ ]	[ ]	[ ]	[ ]	[ ]
Breakfast					
Mid-morning					
Lunch					
Mid-afternoon					
Dinner					
Evening					
Total Units Eaten:	[ ]	[ ]	[ ]	[ ]	[ ]

Tips on Following the Weight Loss Plan

The anti-hypertensive diet is designed to be as flexible as possible, so it should fit into everyone's lifestyle – whether or not you need to lose weight.

You don't need recipes or complicated food preparation methods. All you need do is select the amount of food you want to eat per day, within your unit range. Then it is up to you how you prepare and cook your food.

Each day, select your ideal number of units from each food group depending on how much exercise you plan to take. If active, stick to the top end of the unit range. If planning a low-key, restful day – or if your weight loss has slowed – stick to the bottom end of your unit range.

Combine your unit allowances in any way you like to make up your daily menus.

Choose a variety of foods during the week.

Use low-fat yoghurt or fromage frais with herbs, tomato juice, orange/lemon juice and black pepper, etc. as low-fat dressing or sauce for salads, fish and meats.

There are some preferred preparation and cooking methods which reduce the amount of fat you eat overall, and increase the nutrient value of your food. These include:

- eating fruit and vegetables raw or only lightly steamed
- grilling food with only a light brushing of olive or rapeseed oil
- baking
- steaming
- boiling with only minimal amounts of water and no added salt or bicarbonate of soda
- poaching in vegetable stock
- dry- (stir-)frying using a light brushing of olive or rapeseed oil
- If roasting meat, place the meat on a rack within the roasting pan so all the juices and fats drain away.
- When roasting chicken, use a glass funnel roaster onto which you prop the chicken vertically in the oven. All the fats will then drain off so you are left with beautifully flavoured, low-fat meat.
- When making gravy to go with the roast, ensure it is low-fat and nutrient-rich by using gravy granules plus the water your vegetables were cooked in.

Tips to Help You Eat Less

- Drink a large glass of sparkling mineral water before every meal – this will make you feel full more quickly so you eat less.

- If possible, try to eat the main meal of the day at lunchtime – your metabolic rate is higher than in the evening, so more calories are burned than converted into fat. Try not to eat after 8 p.m. at night
- Always sit down at a laid table – don't eat while standing up.
- Serve smaller helpings than you think you need.
- Use a smaller plate than usual.
- Eat more complex, unrefined carbohydrates (such as brown rice, wholegrain cereals, wholemeal bread, wholewheat pasta, etc.) – these contain complex carbohydrates that trigger release of serotonin in the brain which makes you feel fuller more quickly.
- Eat as slowly as possible, so that metabolic messages that you are full, start to come through before you have finished your meal.
    - Chew each mouthful longer than usual.
    - Pause regularly while eating and put down your knife and fork between bites.
    - Re-discover the art of mealtime conversation.
- Concentrate on enjoying your food. Don't read or watch TV at the same time – you will swallow mechanically without appreciating your food – and end up eating more.
- Try not to eat while driving – this can become a bad habit on long journeys.
- Use low-calorie versions of everything possible when cooking or eating. Skimmed milk has almost 50 per cent fewer calories per pint than whole milk. On a half-pint per day allowance, you can save 450 calories a week.
- Cut down on cooking fats. Don't roast or deep fry.
- Low-fat yoghurt is an ideal substitute for cream in most recipes. *NB:* It will curdle if you let it boil.
- When you feel the urge to eat between meals, do some vigorous exercise and work up a sweat – or try cleaning your teeth with strong, tingling toothpaste.
- Keep a food diary and write down everything you eat if the scales refuse to budge.

The Health Benefits of Exercise

One of the most successful lifestyle changes you can make to lower your BP is to increase the amount of exercise you take. This can lower your diastolic BP by around 10 mmHg – similar to the effect of most anti-hypertensive drugs. Taking regular exercise can also benefit several other factors linked with increased risk of high blood pressure and CHD and, as a result, can prolong your life. A study of more than 10,000 men found that exercise reduced the number of age-related deaths from all causes by almost a quarter – even if exercise was not started until middle age. Deaths from CHD were reduced by 41 per cent, independent of other risk factors such as overweight, high blood pressure or smoking cigarettes.

As well as reducing your risk of high blood pressure, exercise can:

- reduce your risk of a stroke by up to 50 per cent
- reduce your risk of diabetes by up to 40 per cent
- reduce your risk of cancer of the colon, rectum or womb by up to a quarter
- reduce high blood cholesterol levels
- reduce your risk of an intestinal haemorrhage
- help to prevent osteoporosis
- help you to maintain a healthy weight
- improve your strength, stamina and suppleness
- stimulate your bowels and keep them regular
- reduce anxiety and tension
- improve your quality of sleep.

Unfortunately, however, according to the British Heart Foundation the average level of physical activity in the UK is low: seven out of ten men and eight out of ten women do not take enough exercise to reduce their risk of heart attack. Only 10 per cent of men and 3 per cent of women reach recommended targets of exercising 20–30 minutes, three times per week. The Medical Research Council recently reported that many Britons are overweight not because they eat too much, but because they are essentially lazy:

- only 20 per cent of men and 10 per cent of women are employed in active occupations
- over a third of adults take less than 20 minutes of moderate activity each week
- less than half ever participate in active sports
- less than a fifth of adults walk continuously for two miles or more per month
- less than a tenth ever use a bicycle
- an average 26 hours a week is spent watching television.

High Blood Pressure and Sex

Many people with hypertension worry about having sex, as they have heard that this puts blood pressure up. It does – but only momentarily, and does not send it any higher than normal exercise, which is beneficial. You can therefore carry on with a normal sex life.

Why Exercise Protects Against CHD

The risk of CHD is almost twice as high in inactive males as in those who are physically active. Exercise protects the heart in a number of ways. It lowers harmful blood cholesterol levels, lowers blood pressure, reduces hardening and furring up of the arteries and also improves the circulation of blood to the heart through small, collateral arteries.

The effect on blood fats is quite marked. In one study, volunteers were fed a high-fat meal of cereal, fruit and cream which provided 66 per cent of calories in the form of fat. Blood samples were taken at regular intervals over the next six hours and blood fat levels analysed. When the subjects indulged in a prolonged bout of brisk walking, their blood fat levels rose much less than usual. This effect was noticed when exercise was taken as much as 15 hours before the meal, and when exercise was taken 90 minutes after the meal.

Perhaps the most striking example of how exercise affects blood fats was shown by Sir Ranulph Fiennes and Dr Michael Stroud during their epic, unassisted journey across the Antarctic in 1992. They needed to eat a high-fat diet to provide as much energy as possible without increasing the weight of their rations. Despite eating over 5,500 kcals a day, and twice as much fat as recommended, they burned most of it off. Their total blood cholesterol levels did not rise, but interestingly their level of beneficial HDL-cholesterol, which protects against CHD, went up while their level of harmful LDL-cholesterol went down. There's no doubt about it: Exercise does good things to your blood fats as far as your heart is concerned – however healthy your diet. If you suffer from hypertension, you should consider starting a gentle, regular exercise programme.

You Don't Have to Overdo It

The World Health Organization suggests that people in good health should exercise strenuously for 20 minutes a day unless they are engaged in heavy manual labour. However, lesser degrees of exercise are still beneficial – and preferable for those who are just starting their fitness regime or who suffer from heart problems or high blood pressure. A realistic exercise level of 20 minutes' brisk exercise three times a week – and probably every day can be enough to lower high blood pressure significantly, but you need to increase your pulse rate to 110–120 per minute and work up a light sweat.

Heart specialists in Australia followed 500 men who took either light exercise on a bicycle, steps or rowing machine with plenty of rests, or who continuously jogged or walked for 30 minutes. After a year, both groups were declared equally fit during treadmill tests.

Walking briskly (7.2 km/4.5 miles per hour) for 30 minutes burns up 200 calories – enough to lose 450 g/1 lb every two weeks if you take this type of exercise every day.

Strength, Stamina and Suppleness

Exercise improves your strength (building up muscle bulk), your stamina (increasing muscle energy stores) and your suppleness (improving the range of movement of joints and making your ligaments and tendons more flexible).

Different sports have different effects on your strength, stamina and suppleness:

* = Slight effect		** = Beneficial effect	
*** = Very good effect		**** = Excellent effect	

Activity	Stamina	Suppleness	Strength
Aerobics	***	***	**
Athletics	***	**	***
Badminton	**	***	**
Circuit training	***	***	***
Cricket	*	**	*
Cycling	****	**	***
Football	***	***	***
Golf	*	**	*
Jogging	****	**	**
Karate/judo	*	**	*
Rounders	**	*	**
Rowing	***	*	**
Skiing (downhill)	**	**	**
Skipping	***	**	**
Squash	***	***	**
Swimming (hard)	****	****	****
Tennis	**	***	**
Walking (ramble)	**	*	*
(brisk/hill)	***	*	**
Weight training	*	**	****
Yoga	*	***	*

How to Start an Exercise Regime

If you are relatively unfit, don't launch straight into a jogging programme. To achieve fitness, start off slowly and take regular exercise lasting at least 20 minutes, for a minimum of three times a week. Once you have achieved a reasonable level of fitness, you should do more. Your level of exercise should be strenuous enough to raise your pulse to the safe 10-second pulse range for your age (*see below*), to work up a slight sweat and to make you slightly breathless.

It is important to start your exercise programme slowly and carefully. If, after years of inactivity, you suddenly take up jogging or squash, you will be putting your heart under unnecessary strain. People starting an exercise programme too vigorously are likely to tear muscles or ligaments, damage joints and end up stiff, sore and lose motivation. You need to start slowly and increase your exercise levels gently and sensibly as your fitness level improves.

If you are over 50 years of age, and haven't exercised regularly, or if you are under your doctor's care for a health problem, seek permission before you start. This is especially important if you have already had a heart attack. Although gentle exercise will help to improve your health, you must tackle this the right way.

- If you are unfit, start slowly and build up the time and effort you spend on exercise.
- Don't eat a heavy meal within two hours of your exercise programme.
- Stop if you feel dizzy, very short of breath, break into a cold sweat or get any pain.

Exercising Sensibly

If you are under the care of a doctor for a heart problem or for high blood pressure, always consult them first to make sure it is safe for you to start a regular, gentle exercise programme. You may need to adjust the exercise suggestions given below and build up your stamina over a longer period of time. If at any time during exercise you feel dizzy, light-headed, develop chest pain, unusual shortness of breath or feel unwell in any way, stop immediately and seek medical advice.

- Make sure you wear loose clothing and proper footwear specifically designed for the exercise, and use any recommended safety equipment.
- Try to exercise away from traffic and, if you are out at night, wear light colours – better still, fluorescent strips. Avoid isolated areas.
- It is important that you start each exercise period by warming up first with a few simple bends and stretches.
- After you have finished exercising, cool down properly by walking slowly for a few minutes – don't just stop suddenly.

- If you have problems with your joints (such as arthritis) or find it difficult to manage a brisk walk, try a non-weight-bearing form of exercise such as cycling or swimming.

Using Your Pulse Rate

Measuring your pulse rate during exercise will ensure you stay within the safe exercise levels for burning fat and getting fit. Your pulse is most easily felt:

- on the inner side of your wrist on the same side as your thumb (radial pulse)
- at the side of your neck, under the jaw (carotid pulse).

Count your pulse after sitting quietly for around 15 minutes. This is your resting pulse rate. The heart beats approximately 70 times per minute in the averagely fit person.

Resting Pulse Rate (beats per minute)	Level of Fitness
50–59	Excellent (trained athletes)
60–69	Good
70–79	Fair
80 or over	Poor

When exercising, you need to keep your heart working at a safe level. This is most easily done by taking your pulse over 10 seconds, and making sure it stays within the 10-second pulse range for your age, as shown on the following chart.

AGE	10-Second Pulse Range
20	20–27
25	20–26
30	19–25
35	19–25
40	18–24
45	18–23
50	17–23
55	17–22
60	16–21
65	16–21
70	15–20

Take your 10-second pulse every 10 minutes or so during your exercise period. If you are unfit, make sure your pulse stays at the lower end of your 10-second pulse range at first, and slowly work up to the upper end of the range over several weeks.

If at any time your pulse rate goes higher than it should, stop exercising and walk around slowly until your pulse falls. When you restart, take things more easily.

Try taking your pulse 1 minute after stopping exercising, too. The more rapidly your pulse rate falls, the fitter you are. After 10 minutes' rest, your heart rate should fall to below 100 beats per minute. If you are very fit, your pulse will drop by up to 70 beats in 1 minute.

After 20 minutes' exercise, you should feel invigorated rather than exhausted.

WARMING UP

Warming up before exercise is important to:

- warm your body – cold muscles can seize or go into cramp
- stretch your limbs and decrease the risk of tearing a muscle or spraining a ligament
- increase your suppleness and joint mobility
- raise your pulse rate and boost your metabolism to mobilize energy stores
- increase blood flow to your muscles in preparation for extra exertion
- help to get you into the right frame of mind.

You can either march on the spot, getting faster and faster, for 5 minutes, or perform a series of stretches such as those described below. Ideally, do both! Stretch first, then do a 'power march' – bring your knees up high and punch the air in front of you with your arms.

WINDMILLS

Stand comfortably with your feet apart and arms down by your sides. Lift both arms forwards and up, keeping them straight, until they are high above your head. Then spread your arms out sideways and down, to complete the circle. Repeat 10 times.

Then do the reverse, with arms initially going backwards and up. Repeat 10 times.

HEAD ROLLS
Stand comfortably with your feet apart. Place your hands on your hips. Drop your chin to your chest and gently roll your head to the left, back to centre, then to the right, 5–10 times. If this hurts or makes you feel dizzy, stop.

SHOULDER SHRUGS
Stand comfortably, feet apart with your arms by your sides. Lift your shoulders as high as you can and keep them there for a count of 3. Relax. Repeat 10 times.

SHOULDER ROLLS
Stand comfortably with feet apart. Let both arms hang down by your sides. Slowly circle one shoulder forwards, upwards then backwards and downwards. Do this 10 times both sides, getting faster and faster as you go.

SIDE BENDS
Stand comfortably with feet apart and hands by your sides. Slowly bend sideways to your left, so that your left hand travels down the side of your leg as far as is comfortable. Then slowly straighten and repeat on the right hand side. (Don't lean forwards or backwards, but sideways only.) Repeat 10 times to the left then 10 to the right.

TWISTERS
Stand comfortably, feet slightly apart. Link your hands in front of you so your arms are straight out in front of you. Without moving your hips, swivel smoothly to the left, by twisting your waist. When you have twisted as far as you can, hold your position for a count of 3. Return to face front and repeat the twist to the right. Repeat, left then right, 5–10 times.

KNEE BENDS

Stand comfortably, feet slightly apart, by the side of a chair. Rest one hand lightly on the chair back for support. Slowly bend your knees and hips and drop down into a squatting position. Slowly stand up again. Repeat 5–10 times.

VERTICAL TOE TOUCHERS

Stand comfortably, feet slightly apart, arms by your sides. Bend forwards and try to touch your toes. Slowly stand up again. Repeat 5–10 times. If you feel dizzy, stop.

CALF STRETCHES

Stand comfortably, feet apart. With your right foot, take a good step forwards so that your left heel comes up off the ground. Bend your right knee a little and place both hands on your right thigh. Slowly, try pressing your left heel back towards the ground so that you feel your left calf stretching. Hold the stretch for a count of 10. Repeat with the other leg.

THIGH STRETCHES

Stand in front of a wall and, leaning forwards slightly, place your right hand flat against the wall to keep yourself steady. Bend your left knee and bring your left foot up behind you. Grasp your left ankle behind you with your left hand. Pull your ankle in as close to your bottom as you can. Slowly count to 10, then release. Do the same with your right foot and hand.

HORIZONTAL TOE TOUCHERS

Sit on the floor, your legs together in front of you. Reach forwards and try to touch your toes. Hold as far forwards as you can for a count of 10.

HAMSTRING CHEST HUGGERS

Lie on your back. Keeping your bottom on the ground, bend up one knee and clasp both hands behind your thigh. Hug this leg as close to your chest as possible. Allow your other leg to bend too. Hold for a slow count of 10, then repeat with your other second leg.

HAMSTRING STRETCHES

Sit on the floor with legs spread apart. Bend your right knee sideways and bring your right foot up against your left knee. Try to keep your right knee touching the ground. Keeping your left leg straight, slowly bend forwards and try to touch your left ankle or foot. Hold for a count of 10. Repeat with the other leg.

Walking Yourself Fit

Brisk walking is an excellent exercise for building up your cardiovascular fitness level – especially if you've been relatively inactive in recent years. Swing your arms and put as much effort into your walking as possible. Begin slowly and lengthen your strides as you go. You should soon feel warm and start to generate a light sweat. Don't let yourself feel out of breath to the extent that you can't walk and talk at the same time. After your brisk walk, stroll gently for a few minutes to cool down, then do some simple stretching exercises to maintain muscle suppleness.

A suggested walking-for-fitness regime is given below. Obviously you don't need to stick to the days of the week suggested, but try to spread your activity evenly throughout the week. If you find you can comfortably walk briskly for longer than the exercise periods suggested, then increase the time you spend and the distance covered to fast-track your way to fitness and better health.

WEEK	TUESDAY	THURSDAY	SATURDAY	SUNDAY
1	10 MINS	10 MINS	15 MINS	
2	10 MINS	10 MINS	15 MINS	
3	10 MINS	15 MINS	15 MINS	
4	15 MINS	15 MINS	15 MINS	15 MINS
5	15 MINS	15 MINS	20 MINS	20 MINS
6	20 MINS	20 MINS	25 MINS	25 MINS
7	25 MINS	25 MINS	25 MINS	25 MINS
8	30 MINS	30 MINS	30 MINS	30 MINS
9	30 MINS	35 MINS	30 MINS	35 MINS
10	40 MINS	35 MINS	40 MINS	35 MINS
11	40 MINS	40 MINS	40 MINS	40 MINS
12	45 MINS	40 MINS	45 MINS	40 MINS

If at any time you feel you have reached your comfortable exercise level and do not fancy walking any further, then stick at that level. After a while, when you feel like walking further, slowly build up your workout at your own pace.

To maintain your new fitness level, continue walking briskly three or four times a week. Try to take at least 30 minutes' exercise three times per week.

Cycling Yourself Fit

Cycling is an excellent all-round exercise. It is a low-impact, non-weight-bearing aerobic activity which, like swimming, doesn't put your muscles, ligaments or joints under excessive strain. This makes cycling particularly good for the overweight or those with joint problems. Cycling exercises the muscles in your legs, bottom, heart, stomach, lower back, arms and chest.

IN THE GYM

For the averagely non-fit person, start off on an exercise bike using a hill-profile type of programme. A trainer will help you to tailor a cycling regime to suit your fitness goals. A typical one might be as follows:

WEEK	DIFFICULTY LEVEL	VISIT 1	VISIT 2	VISIT 3
1	TWO	6 MINS	6 MINS	6 MINS
2	TWO	6 MINS	6 MINS	6 MINS
3	THREE	6 MINS	6 MINS	6 MINS
4	THREE	12 MINS	12 MINS	12 MINS
5	THREE	12 MINS	12 MINS	18 MINS
6	THREE	18 MINS	18 MINS	18 MINS
7	FOUR	18 MINS	18 MINS	18 MINS
8	FOUR	18 MINS	18 MINS	24 MINS

If at any time you feel you have reached your comfortable exercise level and do not want to increase the difficulty level, or the amount of time you spend on the cycle, then stick at that level. After a while, when that level becomes easier and you feel like increasing the resistance of the bike, or the time you spend on it, slowly build up your workout at your own pace.

If you own your own bike, it is important to be aware of cycling safety:

- Use lights at dusk.
- Fit a red reflector to the rear and amber reflectors to your pedals.
- Maintain and oil your bike regularly.
- Wear reflective clothing at night.
- Avoid roads where there is fast or heavy traffic.
- Consider taking a cycling proficiency test.
- Always wear a safety helmet to BSI 6863 (not for speed cycling or racing) or to American Snell or ANSI standards.

Initially, cycle during the day on a route you know well where there are plenty of other people about and little traffic. Keep to level ground for the first few weeks, then slowly introduce gentle hills. When you feel up to it, try cycling up steeper inclines.

A suggested beginner's cycling regime is given below:

WEEK	TUESDAY	THURSDAY	SATURDAY	SUNDAY
1	15 MINS	15 MINS	15 MINS	
2	15 MINS	15 MINS	15 MINS	
3	20 MINS	20 MINS	20 MINS	
4	20 MINS	20 MINS	20 MINS	20 MINS
5	20 MINS	20 MINS	20 MINS	20 MINS
6	20 MINS	25 MINS	20 MINS	25 MINS
7	25 MINS	25 MINS	25 MINS	25 MINS
8	30 MINS	30 MINS	30 MINS	30 MINS
9	30 MINS	30 MINS	30 MINS	35 MINS
10	35 MINS	35 MINS	35 MINS	35 MINS
11	35 MINS	35 MINS	35 MINS	40 MINS
12	40 MINS	40 MINS	45 MINS	60 MINS

If at any time you feel you have reached your comfortable exercise level and do not fancy cycling further or for longer, stick at that level. After a while, when that level becomes easier and you feel like cycling further or trying a gentle hill, slowly build up your workout at your own pace.

To maintain your new fitness level, continue cycling three or four times per week. Try to average at least three hours of brisk exercise spread out over each seven-day period.

How Many Calories Does Exercise Burn?

To give you an idea of how exercise can help you to lose any excess weight, the following chart shows the calorie-burning value of different forms of exercise:

Activity	Approximate Number of Calories Burned Per Hour
Sitting	90
Standing	100
Driving a car	140
Walk (stroll)	180
Bowling	250
Gardening	250
Swimming	300
Golf	300
Brisk walking	350
Dancing	350
Jogging	500
Tennis	500
Cycling	650

BP AND YOUR DIET

If you suffer from hypertension, it is important to be careful with your diet and to take a few precautions, such as cutting back on salt, eating more of certain fats and less of others, as well as eating plenty of fresh fruit and vegetables for their protective antioxidant content.

Dietary Fats, High Blood Pressure and Atherosclerosis

People with hypertension should pay particular attention to the fats in their diet. By eating more of certain beneficial fats and less of potentially harmful ones, you can help to reduce your risk of future complications such as atherosclerosis, peripheral vascular disease, CHD and stroke.

Fats from your food are processed in your small intestines to form globules (chylomicrons) of fat bound to carrier proteins (to make lipoproteins) which are then absorbed into your bloodstream. After a fatty meal, there may be so many of these fatty particles in your blood that your plasma (blood fluid) takes on a milky white appearance. These chylomicrons are cleared from your bloodstream by the action of an enzyme (lipoprotein lipase) found in the walls of your blood capillaries. Some of the fat released in this way is taken up into cells, while some free fatty acids remain bound to protein and remain in your circulation for transportation to the liver. The fats are then processed, packaged to different types of carrier proteins and passed out into the circulation again for further distribution around your body.

There are two types of circulating cholesterol:

1. low-density lipoprotein (LDL) cholesterol, which is linked with hardening and furring up of artery walls (atherosclerosis), high blood pressure and CHD
2. high-density lipoprotein (HDL) cholesterol, which protects against atherosclerosis and CHD by transporting LDL-cholesterol away from the arteries for metabolism.

It is not your total blood cholesterol level that is important when it comes to atherosclerosis and CHD, but your ratio of LDL- to HDL-cholesterol.

High levels of HDL-cholesterol protect against CHD – because the molecules are too large to seep into artery walls to fur them up, while high levels of LDL-cholesterol increase the risk of atherosclerosis as they are small enough to accumulate in artery walls. Research shows that as your HDL-cholesterol level rises by 1 per cent, your risk of CHD falls by 2 per cent. This seems to be due to reversed cholesterol transport, in which HDL-cholesterol helps to move LDL-cholesterol away from the tissues and back towards the liver.

The Importance of Dietary Fats

If you suffer from hypertension, it is important not to eat too much fat. While a certain amount of fat is important for your health, too much of certain fats is harmful. Ideally you should obtain no more than 30 per cent of your daily calories in the form of fat – unfortunately, for most people in the Western world, their intake averages 40 per cent or more.

The types of fat in your diet is also important. If you ate all your fat in the form of essential fatty acids and fish oils, for example, your risk of CHD would be low, as most circulating fats would be in the form of beneficial HDL-cholesterol.

Eating too much saturated fat has been blamed for overweight and – until recently – was thought to be the main culprit in raising blood cholesterol levels and triggering atherosclerosis. Researchers now increasingly believe that it is eating too many omega-6 polyunsaturated fatty acids (mainly found in vegetable oils) and not enough omega-3 polyunsaturated fatty acids (mainly found in fish oils) that increases your risk of atherosclerosis and other inflammatory diseases such as eczema, asthma, inflammatory bowel disorders and arthritis. This is especially true if your intake of antioxidants (such as vitamins C, E, betacarotene and the mineral selenium) is low. Antioxidants, which are mainly found in fresh fruit and vegetables, help to protect body fats from a chemical alteration known as oxidation. Oxidation produces harmful by-products (such as lipid peroxides) which are now thought to be the cause of a number of common killer diseases, including atherosclerosis, CHD and even cancer.

Types of Fat in Your Diet

Many fats in your diet are made up of a molecule of glycerol to which three fatty acid chains are attached to form a molecular shape similar to that of a capital E (triglycerides). The way your body metabolizes these fats depends on the length of the fatty acid chains and whether or not they contain a chemical joint called a double bond:

- Fats containing no double bonds are called saturated fats.
- Fats containing some double bonds are known as unsaturated fats:
  - Those with two or more double bonds are polyunsaturated fats (PUFAs).
  - Those with one double bond are monounsaturated.

Most dietary fats contain a blend of saturates, monounsaturates and polyunsaturates in varying proportions. In general, saturated fats tend to be solid at room temperature, while monounsaturated and polyunsaturated fats tend to be liquid – that is, oils.

Saturated Fats

Most dietary saturated fats are of animal origin. Coconut is one of the few plant sources of saturated fat.

Until recently, saturated fats were thought to be the main cause of raised blood cholesterol levels. The picture is now less clear-cut. As some experts point out, saturated fat is the form your body preferentially chooses to store its excess calories, which would be unlikely if saturated fats were so harmful.

New research shows that saturated fatty acids containing chains of up to 10 carbon atoms, and in excess of 16 have no effect on blood cholesterol levels. Only saturated fats with carbon chains of 12, 14 and 16 have any reported effect. As a result, over a third of the saturated fats found in animal fats such as milk and butter have no effect on blood cholesterol. In particular, stearic acid (18 carbon atoms) found in milk fat, cocoa butter and meat fat have been found to have no cholesterol-raising activity.

This is backed by data from one of the longest-running studies into CHD, which showed no link between high blood cholesterol levels and saturated fat intake. In fact, analysis of data from the Framingham Heart Study found that, while saturated fat intake increased as a proportion of energy in those studied from 16.4 per cent (1966–69) to 17.0 (1984–88), significant decreases in blood total and LDL-cholesterol levels occurred. For those of normal weight, with no significant family history of high blood cholesterol levels and a good intake of dietary antioxidants, intakes of saturated fat are probably less important than excessive intakes of some polyunsaturated fats.

This is not to say that a high saturated fat intake is not harmful – like all fats, it has a high calorie content and excess is linked with obesity. If you have a family history of atherosclerosis, CHD or high blood cholesterol levels, you may have inherited genes which mean you process saturated fat less well than other people. Some research also suggests that saturated fat intake may contribute to high blood pressure, although the mechanism is unclear. When a group of people cut back on saturated fats, their systolic BP dropped by an average of 7.5 mmHg and diastolic by 2.8 mmHg – even though their intake of sodium chloride (salt) remained the same. When they went back to their previous high saturated fat diet, however, their blood pressures rose to previous levels.

PUFAs

Unlike saturated fats, polyunsaturated fatty acids (PUFAs) have spare double bonds which can make them unstable and highly reactive. Polyunsaturated fats (PUFAs) are of two main types:

1. omega-3 PUFAs
2. omega-6 PUFAs.

Your body handles omega-3 and omega-6 oils in different ways. Omega-3 PUFAs – mainly derived from fish oils – help to counter the stickiness of blood and have beneficial effects on blood cholesterol levels; you should try to eat more of these. Omega-6 PUFAs – mainly derived from vegetable oils – are now thought to be harmful in excess and have been linked with an increased risk of chronic inflammatory diseases such as asthma, auto-immune diseases (such as eczema and rheumatoid arthritis) and some tumours.

Ideally, you need a balanced intake of omega-3s and omega-6s, but the average Western diet currently contains a ratio of omega-6 to omega-3 fats of around 7:1, which is now felt to be far too high.

Omega-3 fish oils contain an essential fatty acid, EPA (eicosapentanoic acid), which is derived from algae eaten throughout a fish's life. Eating fish regularly has a thinning effect on your blood and has been shown to reduce your risk of high blood pressure, heart attack, stroke, inflammatory bowel disease, rheumatoid arthritis and psoriasis. In fact, eating oily fish at least twice a week can lower your risk of CHD more than following a low-fat, high-fibre diet. Research shows that the protective effects of oily fish are seen after only six months; after two years, those on a high fish diet are almost a third less likely to die from CHD than those not eating much fish. This rapid effect is probably due to a thinning effect on the blood, which reduces the chance of blood clots.

EPA has such powerful beneficial effects on health that you should aim to eat at least 300 g of oily fish (such as mackerel, herring, salmon, trout, sardines, pilchards) per week – for most people this means increasing their average fish intake by a factor of 10.

If you are not keen on eating more fish, capsules containing omega-3 fish oils are highly recommended instead. Natural fish oils contain little vitamin E and can go rancid easily. If buying fish oil capsules, choose preparations fortified with vitamin E. Some researchers suggest taking 30–200 iu vitamin E and 50–200 mcg selenium daily as well.

Take fish oils only under strict medical supervision if you:

- have a tendency to bleed easily, or are taking a blood-thinning agent such as warfarin
- have diabetes: several research groups have found that fish oils may increase blood sugar levels and lower insulin secretion in patients with diabetes of both type I and type II categories. These adverse metabolic effects are reversible when supplements are discontinued, but no diabetes sufferer should take fish oil supplements except with the knowledge, consent and monitoring of his or her GP.

TRANS-FATTY ACIDS

When polyunsaturated oils are partially hydrogenated to solidify them in the production of cooking fats and spreads (such as margarine), some trans-fatty acids (named after their chemical structure) are produced. When trans-fatty acids are incorporated into your cell membranes, they increase their rigidity and also seem to raise blood levels of LDL-cholesterol and to lower HDL-cholesterol levels. Trans-fatty acids have therefore been linked with an increased risk of atherosclerosis, high blood pressure, CHD and stroke.

Most people consume around 5–7 g of dietary trans-fatty acids per day. Some people eat as much as 25–30 g of trans-fatty acids a day, particularly if they use cheap margarines and eat lots of processed foods. Researchers have raised so many concerns about the safety of trans-fatty acids that some margarines and low-fat spreads have been reformulated. In Denmark, for example, new guidelines aim to reduce intakes of trans-fatty acids from margarine from 5 g/day to no more than 2 g/day.

Trans-fatty acids are also produced in the rumen of cattle, sheep and goats, so that small amounts (2–4 per cent) are found in dairy products and meat. These naturally occurring trans-fats are structurally different from those released during the commercial hydrogenation of fats, and have so far not been shown to increase the risk of CHD. This has stirred up the butter *vs* margarine controversy, in that some scientists now believe that it is healthier to eat butter than margarine or low-fat spreads. The best advice is to eat as wide a variety of foods as possible, including a little of everything (i.e., both butter and margarine) and to eat nothing to excess.

ESSENTIAL FATTY ACIDS

The essential fatty acids (EFAs) cannot be synthesized in your body from other dietary fats and must therefore come from your food. There are two EFAs:

1. linoleic acid – an omega-6 PUFA
2. linolenic acid – an omega-3 PUFA

A third fatty acid, arachidonic acid – an omega-6 PUFA – may be essential if supplies of other EFAs (from which it can be made in the body) are low.

Unfortunately, as many as 8 out of 10 people do not get enough EFAs from their diet. In addition, the metabolic pathways through which your body converts one EFA into another are easily blocked by lifestyle factors such as eating or drinking too much saturated fat, sugar or alcohol, lack of vitamins and minerals, smoking cigarettes and being under excessive stress.

EFAs are important because they act as building blocks for fatty structures in your body, including those found in your cell membranes and arterial walls. If your intake of EFAs is low, your body can use the next best fats available (such as saturated fats, omega-6 PUFAs, trans-fats) and incorporate them into your cell walls. This can affect the elasticity and quality of your arteries, making them more prone to damage from high blood pressure and atherosclerosis. EFAs also act as building blocks for hormones and hormone-like chemicals called prostaglandins. Lack of EFAs has therefore been linked with a wide range of health problems, from dry, itchy or inflamed skin to hormonal problems such as acne, prostate problems and low sex drive.

EFAs are found in nuts, seeds, green leafy vegetables, oily fish, wholegrains and supplements such as Evening Primrose Oil. Evening Primrose Oil (EPO) supplements are a rich source of gamma-linolenic acid and help to overcome lack of dietary EFAs. Scientists have found that EPO is useful in treating high blood pressure, high cholesterol levels, irritable bowel syndrome, rheumatoid arthritis, eczema and psoriasis.

DIETARY SOURCES OF ESSENTIAL FATTY ACIDS

- Linoleic acid is found in sunflower seeds, almonds, corn, sesame seeds, pumpkin seeds, safflower oil and extra virgin olive oil.
- Linolenic acid is found in Evening Primrose Oil, starflower (borage) seed oil and blackcurrant seed oil.
- Both linoleic and linolenic acids are found in rich quantities in walnuts, soybeans, linseed oil, rapeseed oil and flax oil.
- Arachidonic acid is found in many foods (such as seafood, meat, dairy products) and can also be made in the body from linoleic or linolenic acids.

Monounsaturated Fats

Monounsaturated fats consist of chains of carbon atoms in which there is only one double (unsaturated) bond. This type of fat has largely been ignored by dietary recommendations and there is no specific advice relating to how much you should consume. This is surprising, given that monounsaturates are not susceptible to oxidation and are metabolized in such a way that they lower LDL-cholesterol levels with no effect on HDL levels. A diet high in monounsaturated fats may help to reduce your risk of atherosclerosis, high blood pressure, CHD and stroke. Eating more monounsaturates in place of omega-6 PUFAs would help to reduce the risk of CHD as well as bringing the dietary ratio of omega-3s and omega-6s into a better balance. This is thought to explain some of the benefits of the so-called Mediterranean diet. Foods rich in monounsaturates include olive oil, rapeseed oil and avocado.

Antioxidants and Dietary Fats

Some researchers now believe that even high levels of LDL-cholesterol may not be too harmful as long as your intake of antioxidants is adequate. Antioxidants are substances that help to prevent potentially harmful chemical changes (oxidation) occurring throughout the body. If circulating fats (especially LDL-cholesterol and omega-6 PUFA) are oxidized, they become damaged and attract the attention of scavenger cells (macrophages – *see page 43*). These cells attack the oxidized fats – perhaps mistaking them for foreign invaders such as bacteria – with powerful chemicals. This triggers inflammation at the site of the attack – in or on artery walls – and hastens the hardening and furring up process. Some experts now feel that eating more antioxidants can protect against atherosclerosis, high blood pressure and stroke. Several vitamins and minerals act as antioxidants. The most important are:

- vitamin A and betacarotene
- vitamin C
- vitamin E
- selenium.

Lesser antioxidants which also play a role include:

- riboflavin
- copper
- manganese
- zinc.

FREE RADICALS

Most harmful oxidation reactions occurring throughout the body are caused by free radicals. These are highly reactive molecular fragments produced as a by-product of many metabolic reactions. They only exist momentarily as they carry an electrical charge which they are desperate to off-load. They do this by bombarding your cellular structures, including the nucleus and genetic material, to pinch an electrical charge which neutralizes their own. This can trigger a cascade of damaging reactions linked with atherosclerosis, premature ageing, inflammatory diseases and even cancer. Dietary antioxidants provide your main protection against metabolic free radicals, but unfortunately, many people do not eat enough of them.

What to Do If You Have Hypertension

It now seems that low HDL-cholesterol is a more consistent risk factor for atherosclerosis, CHD and stroke than high LDL-cholesterol, especially in women.

If you are told you have a raised blood cholesterol level, it is important to know whether your LDL- or HDL-cholesterol is high:

- If your blood fats consist mainly of HDL-cholesterol, your risk of CHD is significantly reduced.
- If most of the lipids are in the form of LDL-cholesterol, your risk of CHD is significantly increased.

If your circulating levels of triglycerides – fats containing glycerol attached to three fatty acid chains – are raised, your risk of CHD is also increased.

Your blood fat levels are best measured first thing in the morning after your overnight fast, before you eat or drink anything. This is because your triglyceride levels increase during digestion of dietary fats.

Classification of Total Blood Cholesterol Levels

Desirable	less than 5.2 mmol/l
Borderline	5.2–6.4 mmol/l
Abnormal	6.5–7.8 mmol/l
High	higher than 7.8 mmol/l

Normal Range for Various Blood Lipids

Total cholesterol	less than 5.2 mmol/l
LDL-cholesterol	less than 3.5 mmol/l
HDL-cholesterol	higher than 1 mmol/l
Triglycerides	less than 2.3 mmol/l

Slightly stricter criteria apply to men under the age of 30 and for all patients with CHD.

Studies suggest that 27 per cent of men and 32 per cent of women in the UK have blood cholesterol levels above 6.5 mmol/l (abnormal).

It is estimated that a rise in blood cholesterol of just 1 per cent increases the risk of CHD by 3 per cent. By reducing the average blood cholesterol level by 10 per cent, over a quarter of CHD deaths in the UK could be prevented.

If you suffer from high blood pressure, you can help to reduce your risk of atherosclerosis, CHD and stroke by manipulating your dietary fats so that the ratio between your HDL-cholesterol and LDL-cholesterol levels increases:

- Reduce your overall consumption of fat so that it makes up no more than 30 per cent of your daily energy intake – with saturated fat ideally making up no more than 15 per cent of daily calories.
- Eat more monounsaturated fats (such as virgin or extra virgin olive oil).
- Reduce your intake of omega-6 fatty acids (mainly found in vegetable oils) and increase your intake of omega-3 fatty acids (mainly found in fish oils).
- Eat as few processed foods as possible to reduce your intake of trans-fatty acids.

Other Important Dietary Factors for People with Hypertension

Salt Sensitivity

Research suggests that at least 1 in 2 people is genetically pro-grammed to develop high blood pressure if salt (sodium chlo-ride) intake is excessive. Although not everyone is sensitive to this effect of salt intake, it is worth cutting back on salt if you suffer from hypertension – new data (from the Intersalt study involving 10,000 people in 32 countries) suggests that the link between salt intake and rising blood pressure with increasing age may be stronger than previously thought. Try following a low-salt diet for a month, then have your BP rechecked to see if it has made any difference. If you suffer from kidney problems as well as hypertension you should definitely follow a low-salt diet, as you may not be able to excrete as much salt as normal-ly so that it builds up in your body and contributes to your blood pressure problem. New research suggests that people with the highest blood levels of the kidney hormone renin are most likely to respond to following a low-sodium, high-potassium diet. This research is currently being investigated further. In the mean time, everyone with high blood pressure should consider altering his or her salt intake.

Ideally, you should obtain between 4–6 g salt per day. Aver-age intakes are 6 g per day, however, with some people eating as much as 12 g salt daily. Reducing salt intake by 3 g per day from 9 to 6 g (current UK government recommendations) is estimated to lower your risk of a stroke by 22 per cent and your risk of death from CHD by 16 per cent. Unfortunately, most dietary salt (around 75 per cent) is 'hidden', added to processed foods including tinned products, ready-prepared meals, biscuits, cakes and breakfast cereals. This means that without checking labels and avoiding those products containing high amounts of salt, it is difficult to influence your salt intake as much as is desirable to reduce your risk of hypertension.

To cut back on salt intake, avoid:

- adding salt during cooking or at the table
- salty foods such as crisps, bacon, salted nuts
- tinned products, especially those in brine

- cured, smoked or pickled fish/meats
- meat pastes, pâtés
- ready-prepared meals
- packet soups and sauces
- stock cubes and yeast extracts.

Studies suggest that not adding salt during cooking or at the table will lower your systolic blood pressure by at least 5 mmHg. If everyone did this, it is estimated that the incidence of stroke in the population would be reduced by as much as 26 per cent, and of CHD by 15 per cent.

Salt is easily replaced with herbs and spices as it doesn't take long to retrain your taste buds.

Low Potassium Intake

Dietary potassium helps to flush excess sodium from the body through the kidneys. A diet that is low in potassium has been independently linked with an increased risk of high blood pressure and stroke – especially if your diet is also high in sodium. In one study, people taking anti-hypertensive medication were able to reduce their dose by half (under medical supervision) after increasing the potassium content of their food. To increase your potassium intake, eat more:

- seafood
- fresh fruit, especially bananas, dried apricots, pears and tomatoes
- fruit juices and fruit yoghurts
- vegetables, especially mushrooms, potatoes, aubergines, peppers, squash and spinach
- pulses such as peas and lima beans
- wholegrain breakfast cereals (check labels for sodium chloride content).

Low-salt products containing potassium chloride to replace sodium chloride are popular, but can taste bitter. Too much potassium can unfortunately be harmful, too, so the best way to ensure adequate but safe supplies is to eat potassium-rich foods. Steam rather than boil vegetables to retain more of their mineral content – or if you do cook them in water, make gravy or a low-fat sauce with the cooking water afterwards.

Calcium Intake

The human body contains more calcium than any other mineral. Ninety-nine per cent (around 1.2 kg) is stored in the skeleton, while the other 1 per cent (around 10 g) plays a central role in muscle contraction, nerve conduction, blood clotting, the regulation of metabolic enzymes, energy production and the smooth functioning of the immune system.

The EC recommended daily intake for calcium is 800 mg per day, although to prevent osteoporosis, some people need a daily intake of 1,000–1,500 g per day. Low intakes of calcium have been linked with an increased risk of high blood pressure and stroke. In fact, drugs that affect calcium channels in the body are highly successful in treating hypertension, angina, some irregular heart rhythms and poor circulation (*see page 73*).

Calcium is absorbed in the small intestine, a process for which vitamin D is essential. Usually, less than 40 per cent of dietary calcium is absorbed from the gut – the remainder is lost in bowel motions. Some types of fibre (phytates from wheat in unleavened bread such as chapatti) bind calcium in the bowel to form an insoluble salt that cannot be absorbed. High-fibre diets, which speed the passage of food through the bowels, also reduce the amount of calcium absorbed. As a high-fibre diet is important for health (*see below*) you need to ensure a good intake of calcium – even if this means taking supplements. Some experts recommend that someone with high blood pressure should consider taking a 1,000-mg calcium supplement (plus magnesium, *see below*) with the evening meal (when calcium flux in your body is greatest) for two months to see if this produces a fall in BP.

Symptoms that may be due to calcium deficiency include:

- muscle aches and pains
- muscle twitching and spasm
- muscle cramps
- palpitations
- receding gums.

Foods containing calcium include:

- milk (semi-skimmed and skimmed milks actually contain slightly more calcium than full-fat and are better for your overall health)
- dairy products such as low-fat cheese, yoghurt, fromage frais
- green leafy vegetables such as broccoli
- salmon
- nuts and seeds
- pulses
- white and brown bread – in the UK, white and brown flour (but not wholemeal flour) are fortified with calcium by law
- eggs.

Magnesium

Magnesium and calcium work together in the body; low intakes of magnesium have also been linked with an increased risk of high blood pressure and stroke.

Seventy per cent of your body magnesium is stored in your bones and teeth, but its most important role is to maintain the integrity of your cells. Special salt-pumps maintain different ion concentration gradients across cell walls – these are essential for the cell to act like a battery, holding an electric charge and passing electrical messages from one cell to another. Magnesium is essential for these membrane pumps and for maintaining each cell's electrical stability. It is especially important in controlling calcium entry into heart cells to trigger a regular heart beat.

Magnesium is vital for every major metabolic reaction, from the synthesis of protein and genetic material to the production of energy from glucose. Few enzymes can work without it and magnesium is now known to be vital for healthy tissues, especially those of the muscles, lung airways, blood vessels and nerves. Researchers have found that people with low levels of magnesium are more at risk of spasm of the coronary arteries (linked with angina or heart attack) and spasm of airways leading to asthma, as well as high blood pressure.

The EC recommended daily intake for magnesium is 300 mg. Symptoms that may be due to magnesium deficiency include:

- loss of appetite
- nausea
- fatigue
- weakness
- muscle trembling
- muscle cramps
- numbness and tingling
- loss of co-ordination
- pre-menstrual syndrome
- diarrhoea (early on in deficiency)
- constipation (later on)
- confusion
- nervousness
- insomnia
- palpitations
- dizziness
- hyperactivity
- low blood sugar
- difficult or painful swallowing.

Foods containing magnesium include:

- soya beans
- nuts
- Brewer's yeast
- wholewheat flower
- brown rice
- seafood
- seaweed
- meat
- eggs
- milk
- dairy products
- wholegrains
- bananas
- dark green leafy vegetables
- chocolate
- drinking water in hard-water areas.

Food processing removes most of the magnesium content from these foods, however.

Vitamin C

People with hypertension tend to have a lower blood level of vitamin C than those with normal BP. They also eat less vitamin C, which reflects the link between poor diet and increased risk of atherosclerosis and CHD. New research also confirms that elderly people whose diet is poor in vitamin C are more likely to die of a stroke. This makes sense when you consider that vitamin C is needed in the body for the manufacture of collagen – an important structural protein that strengthens and repairs weak or damaged blood vessels. Vitamin C is also an important dietary antioxidant that can protect against atherosclerosis, CHD, chronic inflammatory diseases and even cancer. The EC recommended daily intake is 60 mg per day to keep your health ticking over. For optimum nutrition, more and more experts now recommend intakes much higher than this. Taking vitamin C supplements have been shown to reduce high BP – try taking 1–3 g vitamin C per day. If taking supplements, it is also worth complementing them with other antioxidants such as vitamin E and betacarotene.

- The risk of developing angina is up to three times lower in people with high blood levels of vitamins E, C and betacarotene.
- Those who have a high intake of vitamin C (including the use of supplements) have up to a 40 per cent lower risk of CHD and a 35 per cent less risk of dying from it.
- People with the highest intakes of betacarotene reduce their risk of CHD by 22 per cent for women, 25 per cent for men.
- Taking vitamin E supplements can reduce the risk of CHD by 12 per cent; in one study, middle-aged males who took them for more than two years reduced their risk by a total of 25 per cent. There are unconfirmed reports that vitamin E may cause a rise in BP in people with very high blood pressure, however.

Co-enzyme Q

Co-enzyme Q is a vitamin-like substance important for the release of energy in cells. It forms part of the system which passes electrons from one molecule to another in mitochondria – small structures inside each cell which act as energy factories. It is also believed to improve the function of blood vessel walls and to regulate blood pressure. Researchers have found that supplements containing co-enzyme Q improve heart muscle function, and it has successfully been used to treat CHD and heart failure. Those with hypertension may be deficient in co-enzyme Q. In one study, people with high blood pressure who took supplements had a significant fall in BP – systolic pressure dropped by an average of 10.6 mmHg, and diastolic pressure by 7.7 mmHg over a period of 10 weeks. Supplements of 60–100 mg per day are worth trying to see if they help.

Fibre

Dietary fibre – or roughage – is a broad term used to describe the indigestible parts of plant foods such as cellulose, hemicellulose, lignin, pectins and gums. Humans lack the enzymes necessary to break down this dietary fibre and release its energy, although bacteria in your gut can ferment them, releasing acids and gases in the large bowel (colon).

Ideally, you need to eat at least 30 g fibre per day. Although this roughage provides little in the way of energy or nutrients, it is essential for helping the digestion and absorption of other foods. Fibre encourages the muscular, wave-like bowel contractions (peristalsis) that propel digested food through the intestines. This regulates bowel function, and also acts like a sponge to absorb water, toxins and bacteria. Research also suggests that dietary fibre absorbs fats and sugars in the bowel and helps to lower blood glucose and cholesterol levels by increasing the amount of fat that is excreted rather than absorbed.

A low-fibre diet is linked with an increased risk of hypertension as well as a number of other diseases, including bowel cancer. Increasing your fibre intake has been shown to lower a high BP. Try to eat more unrefined complex carbohydrates such as wholegrain cereals, wholewheat pasta, wholemeal bread, nuts, fresh fruit and vegetables.

Bran-containing breakfast cereals provide one of the highest concentrations of dietary fibre:

- bran provides 40 g fibre per 100 g portion
- dried apricots 18 g per 100 g
- peas 5 g per 100 g
- prunes 13 g per 100 g
- cooked brown rice 4 g per 100 g
- cooked wholemeal spaghetti 4 g per 100 g
- brown bread 6 g per 100 g
- walnuts 6 g per 100 g.

Vegetarians have a lower blood pressure than most meat-eaters, with BP becoming lower the longer they have avoided meat. Although vegetarians are more likely to have a healthier lifestyle (that is, more likely to take exercise and least likely to smoke), one of the main reasons for their lower BP is their high-fibre, low-fat diet.

Garlic

Garlic cloves contain a natural substance, allicin, which has a powerful protective effect against CHD. Research shows it can:

- lower blood pressure enough to reduce the risk of a stroke by up to 40 per cent
- reduce the risk of CHD by up to 25 per cent
- lower harmful LDL-cholesterol by 12 per cent
- lower triglycerides by 13 per cent
- improve circulation to the skin by 48 per cent
- decrease the risk of blood clots by increasing clot breakdown (fibrinolysis), decreasing blood stickiness (plasma viscosity), decreasing blood cell clumping (platelet aggregation) and possibly preventing a dangerous heart rhythm (ventricular tachycardia).

Allicin (known chemically as diallyl thiosulphinate) is not found in whole garlic cloves, but is released when the clove is crushed. This brings an enzyme, alliinase, into contact with an amino acid, alliin, to produce allicin. This unfortunately starts to break down once it comes into contact with air and during cooking, so the only reliable way to use garlic to protect against heart disease is to take tablets containing standardized garlic extracts in a concentrated form.

Many studies have shown that garlic powder tablets can reduce high blood pressure. When 600–900 mg are taken daily for up to six months, systolic BP fell by an average of 8 per cent (and up to 17 per cent), while diastolic BP was lowered by an average of 12 per cent (and up to 16 per cent). This reduction occurred gradually, although in some cases did not start until after 2–3 months treatment. This significantly lowers your risk of both CHD and stroke. Garlic is thought to work by a combination of:

- increasing the fluidity of blood and decreasing its stickiness – some of the ingredients in garlic (ajoene, methylallyl trisulphide and dimethyl trisulphide) are as powerful as aspirin in this respect
- relaxing smooth muscle cells in arterial walls and dilating blood vessels (arterioles by an average of 4.2 per cent and venules by 5.9 per cent)
- improving transport of sodium and potassium ions across cell membranes.

All these beneficial effects on the circulation can be demonstrated within five hours of taking a single dose of 600- to 900-mg garlic powder tablets, and wear off over 24 hours.

Dietary Changes for a Healthy Heart

People who follow a Mediterranean-style diet seem to have a 75 per cent lower risk of CHD than those eating a typical Western-style diet. The Mediterranean way of eating is thought to reduce atherosclerosis and high blood pressure because it contains olive oil, antioxidant vitamins, garlic, oily fish, red wine and provides plenty of fibre. To follow this way of eating:

- Eliminate as many processed and pre-packed foods as possible – eat wholefoods high in minerals, vitamins and fibre instead.

- Increase your intake of complex carbohydrates (wholegrain cereals, brown rice, wholemeal pasta, wholegrain bread) to 50–70 per cent of daily calories – most people get less than 40 per cent of daily energy from these sources.
- Increase your intake of fresh fruit, salads and vegetables to at least a pound in weight per day (not counting potatoes). This works out at around five or six portions (such as a glass of unsweetened orange juice with breakfast, a large salad at lunch, two pieces of fruit during the day plus two veg with your evening meal).
- Decrease the amount of fat, especially saturated fat, that you eat. Fats should make up no more than 30 per cent of daily calories. Switch to low-fat products and use more olive oil (or rapeseed oil).
- Decrease the amount of red meat you eat to only once or twice per week. Have more vegetarian meals instead, which include pulses and beans for protein.
- Increase the amount of fish you eat. Try to eat at least 300 g (three portions) of oily fish per week.
- Increase the amount of pulses, nuts and seeds you eat. The World Health Organization recommends an intake of 30 g (1 oz) per day. These are a rich source of essential fatty acids which have beneficial effects on blood cholesterol – walnuts are especially beneficial.
- Reduce the amount of simple sugars and sweets you eat. These are rapidly absorbed and cause sugar swings in the blood. This is linked with an increased risk of diabetes and atherosclerosis.
- Cut right back on the amount of salt you eat. Avoid salty foods such as crisps, bacon, tinned/cured/smoked/pickled fish and meats, meat paste, pâté, ready-prepared meals, tinned vegetables or tuna in brine, tinned or packet soups, sauces, stock cubes and yeast extracts. Don't add salt to food during cooking or at the table. Obtain flavour from herbs, spices and black pepper instead. You will soon get used to low-salt food.

  Think about taking daily food supplements:
  – vitamin C (1–3 g), betacarotene (up to 15 mg per day) and possibly vitamin E (30–200 iu)

- garlic tablets (600–900 mg)
- fish oil capsules (1–2 capsules per day)
- a vitamin and mineral supplement that includes calcium (1,000 mg), magnesium (300 mg) and selenium (50–200 mcg)
- co-enzyme Q (60–100 mg).

USEFUL ADDRESSES

Please send a stamped, self-addressed envelope if writing to an organization for information.

ASH (ACTION ON SMOKING AND HEALTH)
   109 Gloucester Place
   London W1H 4EJ
   0171 935 3519

BRITISH HEART FOUNDATION
   15 Fitzharding Street
   London W1H 4DH
   0171 935 0185

DRINKLINE: THE NATIONAL ALCOHOL HELPLINE
   13–14 West Smithfield
   London EC1A 9DH
   0345 320202

PRE-ECLAMPTIC TOXAEMIA SOCIETY
   Eaton Lodge
   8 Southend Road
   Hockley
   Essex SS5 4QQ
   01702 205088

QUIT (NATIONAL SOCIETY FOR NON-SMOKERS)
Victory House
170 Tottenham Court Road
London W1P 0HA
Quitline (helpline for those wanting to stop smoking):
0171 487 3000

STROKE ASSOCIATION
CHSA House
Whitecross Street
London EC1Y 8JJ
0171 490 7999

Complementary Therapies

BRITISH ACUPUNCTURE ASSOCIATION AND REGISTER
34 Alderney Street
London SW1V 4EU
0171 834 1012
Information leaflets, booklets, register of qualified practitioners

BRITISH HERBAL MEDICINE ASSOCIATION
Sun House
Church Street
Stroud GL5 1JL
01453 751389
Information leaflets, booklets, compendium, telephone advice

BRITISH HOMOEOPATHIC ASSOCIATION
27A Devonshire Street
London W1N 1RJ
0171 935 2163
Leaflets, referral to medically qualified homoeopathic doctors

GENERAL COUNCIL AND REGISTER OF NATUROPATHS
Frazer House
6 Netherall Gardens
London NW3 5RR
0171 435 8728

INTERNATIONAL STRESS MANAGEMENT ASSOCIATION
The Priory Hospital
Priory Lane
London SW15 5JJ
0181 876 8261
Information on stress management and control; leaflets, booklets, counselling

FURTHER READING

Dr Duncan Dymond, *The Jargon-Buster's Guide to Heart Disease* (Metro)

Dr David Lewis and Dr John Storey, *Heart Attack – How to Return to a Full, Healthy and Active Lifestyle* (Thorsons)

Dr Tom Smith, *Heart Attacks: Prevent and Survive* (Sheldon Press)

—, *Living with Angina* (Sheldon Press)

DIET AND LIFESTYLE

Leon Chaitow, *Stress* (Thorsons)

Leonard Mervyn, *Thorsons Complete Guide to Vitamins and Minerals* (Thorsons)

Stephen Terrass, *Stress* (Thorsons)

Dr Melvyn Werbach, *Healing through Nutrition* (Thorsons)

COMPLEMENTARY THERAPIES

David Hoffman, *The Complete Illustrated Holistic Herbal* (Element Books)

Dr Andrew Lockie and Dr Nicola Geddes, *The Complete Guide to Homeopathy* (Dorling Kindersley)

Penelope Ody, *The Herb Society's Complete Medicinal Herbal* (Dorling Kindersley)

The Reader's Digest Family Guide to Alternative Medicine

Norman Shealy (ed.), *The Complete Family Guide to Alternative Medicine* (Element Books)

Valerie Ann Worwood, *The Fragrant Pharmacy* (Bantam Books)

INDEX

Of further interest…

HEART ATTACK

How to return to a full, healthy and active lifestyle

DAVID LEWIS AND DR JOHN STOREY

If you have had a heart attack, here is a unique and practical plan to help you back to full and active health. It is a plan that can also bring you back from the brink of a heart attack if stressful living is causing you concern.

Insufficient exercise and poor diet are well-known as major risk factors in the development of heart disease, but the authors argue that the key to a healthy heart lies in your emotional response to life. They pinpoint as a major contribution to heart disease the addictive qualities of noradrenaline, the self secreted 'anger hormone' which drives so many striving and competitive people in stressful occupations.

Heart Attack provides answers to such questions as:

- Will it happen again?
- What jobs can I safely undertake?
- How much exercise do I need?
- Is it essential to avoid all stress?
- Need there be significant restrictions on diet?
- Is it safe to play a strenuous sport?

HEART DISEASE: QUESTIONS YOU HAVE...ANSWERS YOU NEED

KARLA MORALES

Heart disease is the leading cause of death in the Western world. In the light of this sobering statistic, it is essential to know as much as possible about your heart.

This vital guide cuts through the medical jargon and gives clear answers to hundreds of commonly asked questions:

- What causes heart disease?
- What happens during a bypass operation?
- Can heart disease be prevented?
- How dangerous is high blood pressure?
- What is a heart attack?

All the facts you need to know about heart health.

BLOOD PRESSURE: QUESTIONS YOU HAVE...ANSWERS YOU NEED

KARLA MORALES

High blood pressure – hypertension – is one of the most common and most serious of all health conditions.

This vital guide cuts through the medical jargon and clearly answers the most commonly asked questions about high blood pressure, including invaluable advice about how to prevent, and cope with, the disease:

- What causes high blood pressure?
- Can high blood pressure be cured?
- Is it safe to exercise?
- What are the dangers of low blood pressure?
- How does diet affect blood pressure?
- What drugs are used for treatment and how do they work?

RECIPES FOR HEALTH:
HIGH BLOOD PRESSURE

MAGGIE PANNELL

Diet is becoming more and more popular as an effective way of treating, preventing and controlling the development of high blood pressure – hypertension – one of the most common and most serious of all health conditions.

Doctors recommend adopting a diet which is:

- Low in salt
- Calorie-controlled for weight reduction

In this book, Maggie Pannell, an expert on food and nutrition, follows these dietary guidelines and presents delicious ways to reduce blood pressure and eat healthily. She explains the causes and dangers of the condition, suggests which foods to avoid and recommends eating less fat, less sugar and more fibre.

The recipes include exciting ideas for breakfasts, soups and starters, light meals, salads, main meals and desserts as well as a mouth-watering selection of menus for special occasions.

This book can really help to reduce your blood pressure safely – in the most enjoyable way!

HEART ATTACK	0 7225 3227 X	£6.99	☐
HEART DISEASE	0 7225 3312 8	£3.99	☐
BLOOD PRESSURE	0 7225 3314 4	£3.99	☐
RECIPES FOR HEALTH:			
HIGH BLOOD PRESSURE	0 7225 3144 3	£5.99	☐

All these books are available from your local bookseller or can be ordered direct from the publishers.

To order direct just tick the titles you want and fill in the form below:

Name: _____

Address: _____

_____

_____ Postcode: _____

Send to Thorsons Mail Order, Dept 3, HarperCollinsPublishers, Westerhill Road, Bishopbriggs, Glasgow G64 2QT.

Please enclose a cheque or postal order or your authority to debit your Visa/Access account —

Credit card no: _____

Expiry date: _____

Signature: _____

— up to the value of the cover price plus:

UK & BFPO: Add £1.00 for the first book and 25p for each additional book ordered.
Overseas orders including Eire: Please add £2.95 service charge. Books will be sent by surface mail but quotes for air-mail dispatches will be given on request.

24-HOUR TELEPHONE ORDERING SERVICE FOR ACCESS/VISA CARDHOLDERS — TEL: 0141 772 2281.